MISS CRAIG'S
10-MINUTE-A-DAY
SPOT-
REDUCING
PROGRAM

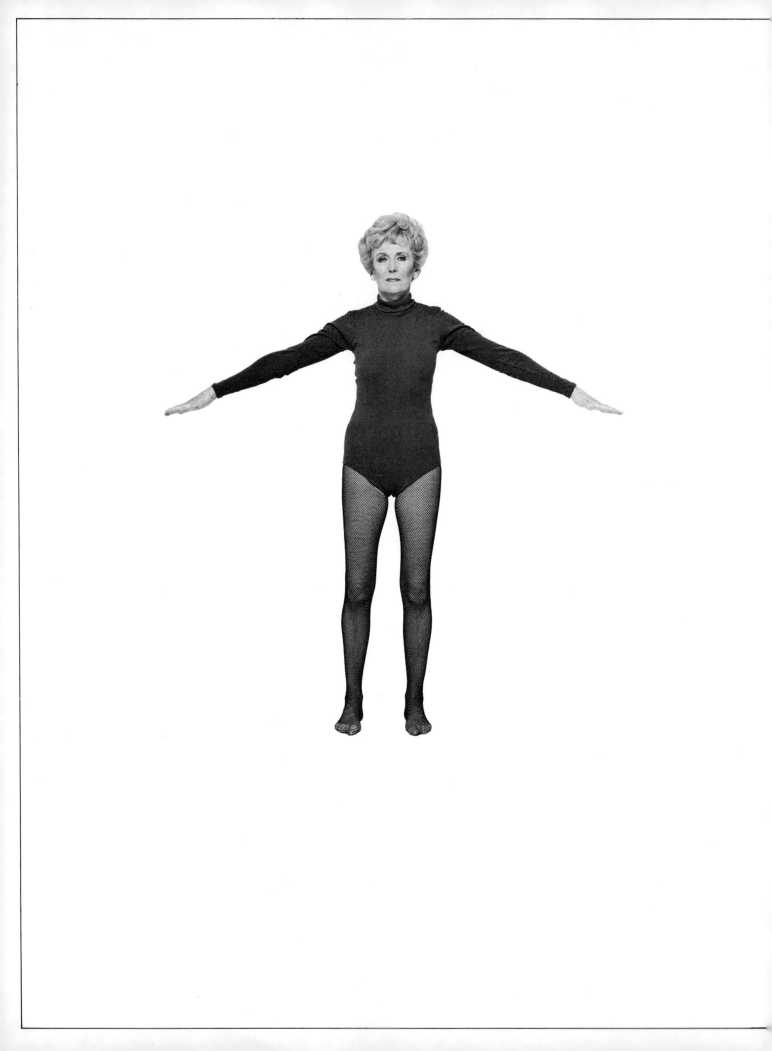

MISS CRAIG'S 10-MINUTE-A-DAY SPOT-REDUCING PROGRAM

A Catalogue of Exercises for Improving Specific Parts of the Body

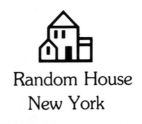

Random House
New York

This book was created under the personal editorship of Phyllis Cerf Wagner

Hair Stylist: Michael Fitzpatrick of Elizabeth Arden
Photographer: Joel Markman
Makeup: Margaret Sunshine
Designer: Robert Aulicino

Library of Congress Cataloging in Publication Data

Craig, Marjorie.
Miss Craig's 10-minute-a-day spot-reducing program.

Includes index.
1. Reducing exercises. I Title. II. Title: 10-
minute-a-day spot-reducing program. III. Title: Spot-
reducing program.
RA781.6.C72   613.7′1   79-4770
ISBN 0-394-50749-5

Manufactured in the United States of America
24689753
First Edition

CONTENTS

For forty-four years—all of my adult life—I have been a teacher of exercises. My training and experience led me to develop a natural-movement exercise program which can be done without the grunts, groans, and contortions, and aches and pains, that one usually associates with getting "in shape." Over the years, this very program has kept my own body trim, as it has those of private clients, and judging from the letters I receive, it has also helped the unseen pupils who learned the exercises from my book Miss Craig's 21-Day Shape-Up Program, which, incidentally, has not been out of print since its publication in 1968. In that book I described, and demonstrated with photographs, a program that when learned takes thirty minutes to perform (which I believe to be the minimum exercise requirement to gain and maintain a healthy-looking and -feeling body) and suggested that it be done every day to get the best results.

My 21-Day Shape-Up Program was designed to tone and firm all the large muscles of the body in a systematic way. If that program works—and I promise you it does—you might properly ask, "Why this book?" The answer: "To fill a different need."

- *It is meant to help those persons who are doing more than thirty minutes of exercise a day (whether that amount of time is spent on the tennis court, the golf course, in the swimming pool, on the ski slopes, on the ice-skating rink or jogging or walking along a city or country road) but who still think they have figure problems and want to do something about them.*

- *It is for those who weigh what they should but who have lumps and bumps and sags where they shouldn't.*

- *It is for those who want to limber up before they run or do some other strenuous exercise.*

- *It is for all of those who are constantly asking me to please give them a good exercise for a potbelly, fat arms, fat thighs, sagging bosoms, a spreading buttocks or waistline—you name it. In other words, it's for anyone looking for a specific exercise to solve a specific figure problem.*

The exercises in this book are different from those in my 21-Day Program, even though all of them are based on exercising muscles with natural move-

ments that will not strain or cause the muscles to ache, but will strengthen, bring tone to and help contour the body. I have not made the changes for change's sake. Toning the entire body can be done much more economically, in terms of time, by involving groups of muscles in a single exercise, and this is the approach I used as I designed the exercises for the 21-Day Program. Spot-reducing, on the other hand—to which the exercises in this book are dedicated—can be done much more rapidly by isolating a specific muscle's movements and giving that muscle a total and thorough workout.

When I started my career as a physical therapist at the Neurological Institute of Columbia Presbyterian Medical Center, I was charged with devising exercises to help rehabilitate the muscles of men, women and children which had been damaged because of illness or accident, or were temporarily weakened by surgery. To give the kind of aid that was needed, it was necessary for me to learn the movements and function of the more than six hundred muscles that make up half of, and control the entire action of, the human body.

The knowledge I gained then—plus the experience I have had subsequently at Richard Hudnut's and for the past twenty-seven years as a teacher of private exercise lessons at Elizabeth Arden's New York Salon and as the Director of the Body Department for all the Arden Salons as well as Maine Chance—led me to understand why one should exercise a muscle "naturally." Gymnastic-type exercises can create muscle strain and/or cause muscle bulge; the former can cause permanent damage to a muscle and the latter can foster restricted movement. While I was testing and evaluating the exercises I have included in the Spot-Reducing Program, I was astounded at how many of my pupils would try a new movement for me, then say, "I'm not sure this exercise is going to do any good—it doesn't hurt when I do it."

Fortunately, the proof that the exercises are good is borne out by the tape measure rather than by how much they hurt.

They work!

In developing these exercises, I have tried, whenever possible, to design them so they can be done by people with limited space. Also, at Elizabeth Arden's, I have my pupils exercise to music, and I suggest you do the same, since muscles seem to respond to it and it makes sessions seem less boring and less tiring.

Though these spot-reducing exercises look deceptively simple, after doing them regularly for just one week, some of my pupils have lost an inch in both their waist and hip measurements.

There is no magic in my method. The person who is going to bring about the difference in you is you. Once you have learned to do the exercises in this program, it should take you no longer than five minutes to do each category. It doesn't matter when you do them, or if you do them all at one time. If you feel like doing them for less than five minutes, you'll still get results—you just won't get them as quickly. If you feel like doing them for more than five minutes, you will not get aching muscles— you'll just see results sooner. Simple as these exercises may seem (and they are), before embarking on any exercise program, you should check first with your doctor.

THE SPOT-REDUCING PROGRAM AND HOW IT WORKS

The program is made up of two segments:

Eight exercises to bring tone systematically to all the large muscles of the body.

Exercises to be picked by categories, i.e., arms, abdomen, thighs, etc., so the exerciser may tailor the program to individual needs.

Both segments can be done—once the exercises have been learned—in just 10 minutes a day.

5 minutes for the 8 general exercises
5 minutes for the spot-reducing exercises

Natural movements are called for in all the exercises, but for spot-reducing, every movement of every muscle as it interacts with other muscles has been considered and programmed in order to bring tone to as many of the fibers as possible.

Without getting too technical, let us simply say that a muscle's tissues are made up of many different fibers. These fibers work in concert to produce a maximum or minimum effort. Professional acrobats and dancers, who train for hours every day, might use all the fibers of the large muscles, but most people do not—and it is this insufficient use which causes muscle fibers to degenerate. This degeneration shows up in the body in the form of lumps and bumps (fat accumulates around lazy muscle tissues), sagging skin (muscles lose elasticity if they are not used often, and so does the skin that covers them) and stiff joints (joints are moved by muscles—

if muscles do not move them, they are apt to become atrophied).

Actually, no muscle works alone; muscles work in pairs and in groups. When one muscle contracts, a partner muscle must extend. Muscles also work in groups to rotate, abduct, adduct and circumduct joints, lift weights, etc. In some instances, "fixing" muscles into set positions gives partner groups greater or less mobility; as an example of this, by "fixing" the knee muscle into a bent position, the thigh may be brought closer to the trunk of the body. The "fixed" principle has been used throughout the spot-reducing exercises to ensure maximum contraction and extension, and thus bring tone more rapidly to those muscles that require "spot" therapy.

GENERAL TONING PROGRAM

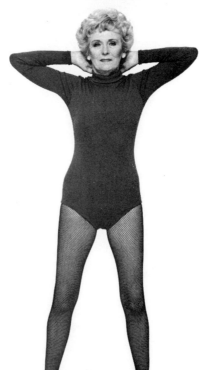

The muscles that generally account for the shapeliness of the total body are those which control the movements of the abdomen, upper back, shoulders, arms, bosom, chest, buttocks, hips, lower back, thighs and waistline. To help the exerciser bring tone to these muscles—and maintain it—I have included, in the Toning Program, one exercise for each of the aforementioned areas.

Unless one is engaged (for at least thirty minutes a day) in active exercises, such as running, skiing, bowling, walking, etc., this program should be done daily as an adjunct to the spot-reducing exercises you have chosen; otherwise, it will be sufficient to do it three days a week.

I suggest to clients that on the days that they skip the Toning Program, they add the time they save to their spot-reducing exercises and do twice the number called for. My theory is, of course, that their spot-reducing will be accomplished just that much faster. I have designated "which" exercises are for "what" in this section to enable you to skip those you do not think you need.

TONING PROGRAM/1

ABDOMEN

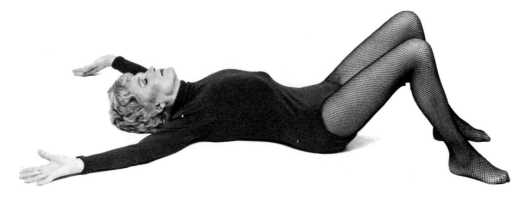

Starting Position: Lie down on your back. Bend knees and place feet flat on the floor. Put arms over your head with elbows firmly on the floor.

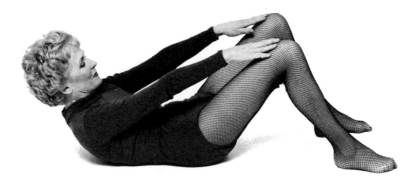

Movements:

1. Raising only head, shoulders and arms, touch hands to knees.

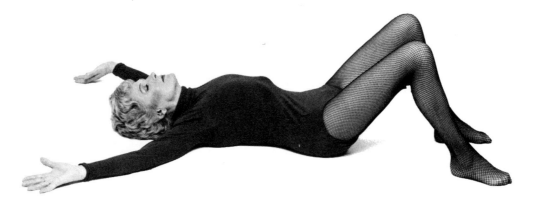

2. Slowly return to starting position.

Do exercise 15 times

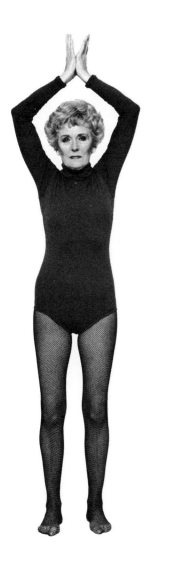
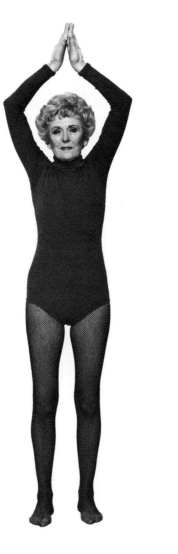
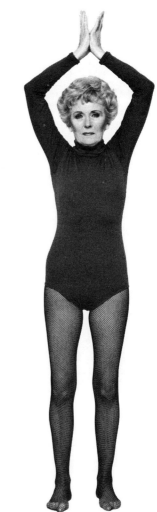

Starting Position:
Stand with arms over your head and the heels of the hands touching.

Movements:
1. Turn your hands until the backs are touching.

2. Return hands to starting position.

Do exercise 30 times: 20 as slowly as possible; 10 quickly.

TONING PROGRAM/3

BACK AND SHOULDERS

Starting Position: Stand with your back pressed against the jamb of a doorway. Bend knees slightly and place feet 16 or more inches from the frame. Bend elbows and grasp the molding behind your head. Keep your back pressed against the jamb throughout this exercise.

Movements:

1. Holding on to the molding with your hands, bring bent arms to your head.

2. Still holding on to the molding, extend bent arms as far as possible away from your head.

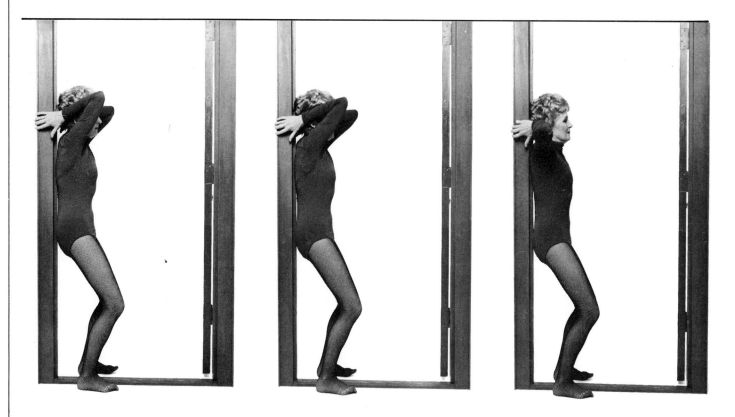

Do exercise 20 times.

BOSOM AND CHEST

Starting Position: Stand at arm's length away from a wall, with both arms extended at shoulder level. Keep arms straight, with one hand pressed against the wall, throughout this exercise.

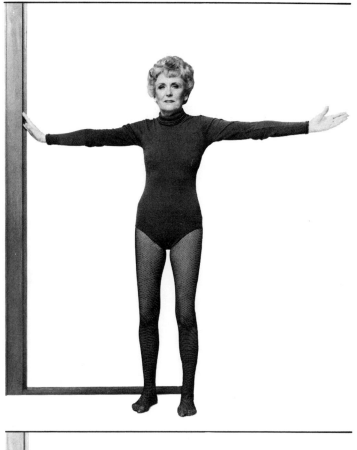

Movements:

Move the left arm across your chest; try to touch the left hand to the right hand 20 times.

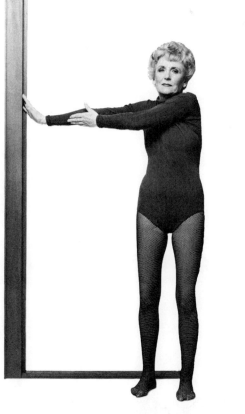

Do exercise 20 times, 10 with each arm.

BUTTOCKS AND HIPS

Starting Position: Stand at the side of a chair, with your right hand resting on it.

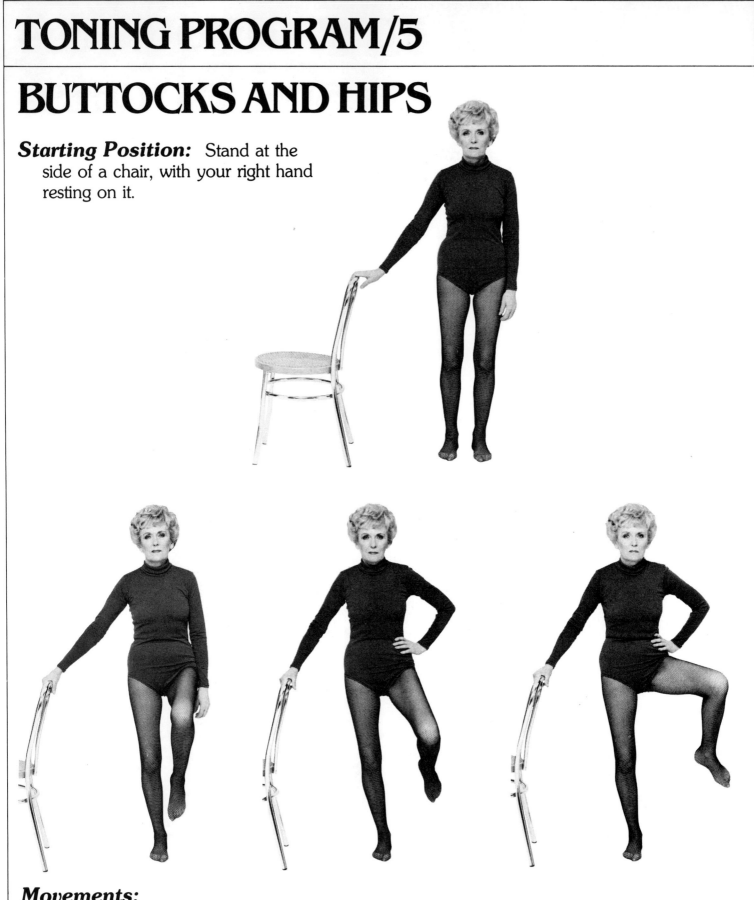

Movements:

1. Raise the left leg about 10 inches, bending your knee in front of you.

2. Circle the leg in this bent position, keeping the foot raised off the floor as you do so. Circle 20 times.

Turn, and circle your right leg 20 times.

LOWER BACK

Starting Position: Bend knees, and leaning over, touch hands to the sides of your feet.

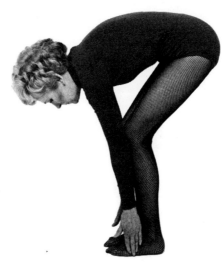

Movements:

1. Keeping your buttocks down and your head tucked into your chest, use the back muscles to slowly raise your body to an upright position.

2. When the body is upright, pinch the shoulder blades together and raise your head to its natural position.

3. Relax the shoulder blades (not the body).

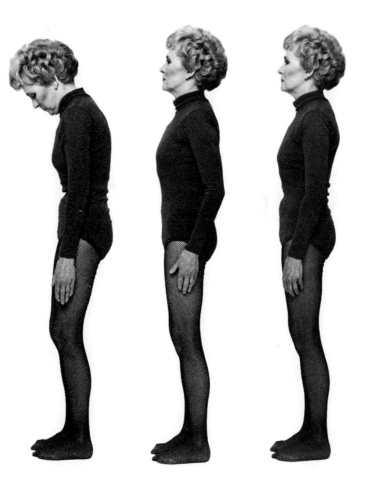

Do exercise 10 times.

THIGHS

Starting Position: Stand with feet about 10 inches apart.

Movements:

1. Keeping feet firmly planted on the floor, shift weight to the right leg. When you've shifted it as far as you think you can, stick your hip out a little farther to the side with three bouncing movements.

2. Return weight to both legs.

3. Shift weight to left leg and repeat movements.

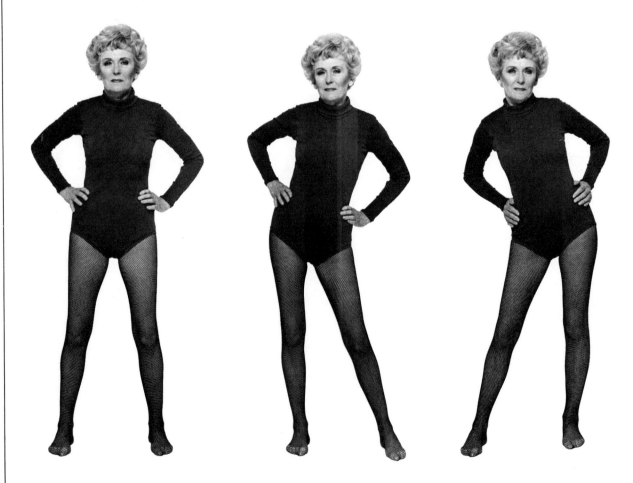

Do exercise 20 times.

WAISTLINE

Starting Position: Stand with knees slightly bent and feet spread apart. Clasp your hands behind your neck.

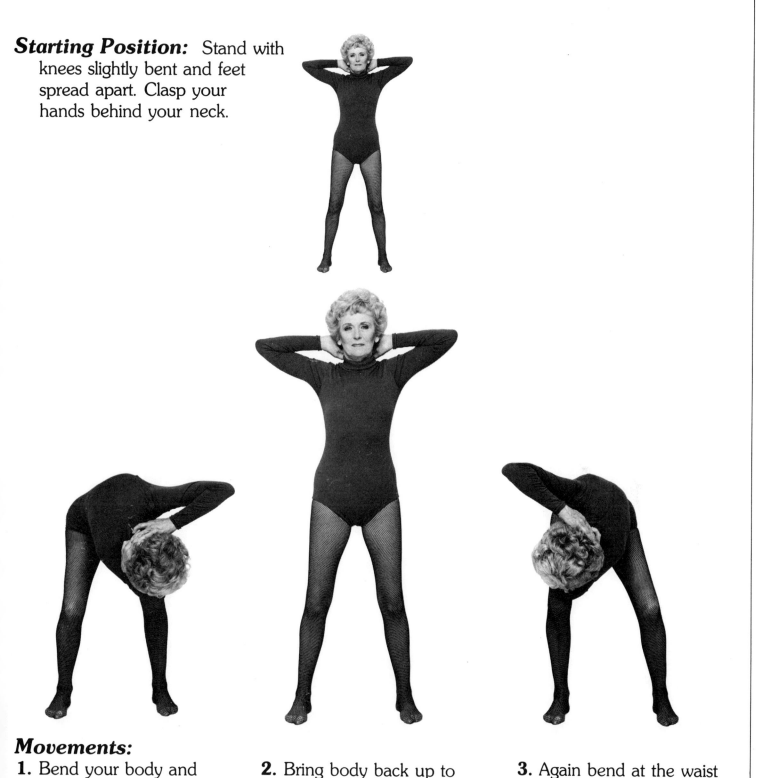

Movements:

1. Bend your body and try to bring the right elbow to the left knee.

2. Bring body back up to a standing position.

3. Again bend at the waist and this time try to bring the left elbow to the right knee.

Do exercise 20 times.

11

SPOT-REDUCING EXERCISES

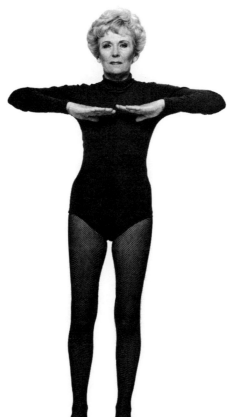

ABDOMEN

The abdominal muscles, acting in concert with the thorax muscles and the diaphragm, not only assist in inspiration and expiration, but in addition, help to bend the trunk of the body forward, rotate the body from side to side, draw the pelvis forward and bend the vertebral column to one side or the other.

Since every little muscle has a movement all its own, one can readily see that the exercise of bending and touching the toes, which is generally given for toning the abdominal muscles, can't possibly do the whole job. Thus, this series of exercises has been divised for firming all the muscles of the abdominal area.

To achieve total firming, it is important to do them all. Though they seem simple (they are, for they are based on natural movements), don't be surprised if at first you find them tiring. It is not necessary to do them all at once, but do do them all sometime every day.

ABDOMEN/1

Starting Position: Sit with knees bent, feet on the floor and arms extended in front of you.

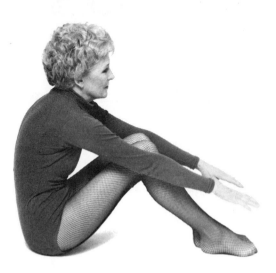

Movements:

1. Slowly lean backward until your hands come about level with your mid-thighs.

2. Hold your body in this lean-back position, with arms still extended, until the abdominal muscles begin to tremble.

3. As soon as these muscles start to tremble, return your body to the starting position.

Do exercise 10 times.

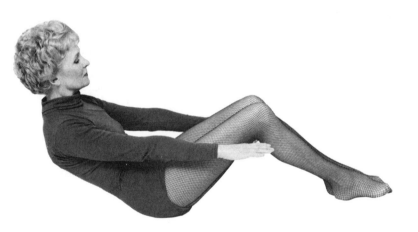

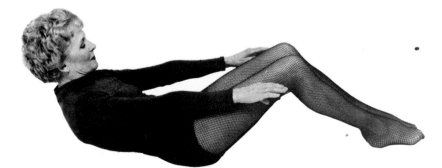

As the abdominal muscles strengthen, lean back farther and farther and hold the lean-back position longer and longer. Try always to return the body to its upright position without touching your head to the floor.

Starting Position: Sit on the floor with arms outstretched at shoulder level and legs extended in front of you. Raise the right leg slightly.

Movements:

1. With right leg raised, twist body and arms to the right as far as you can. Twist 3 times, returning arms to center after each twist.

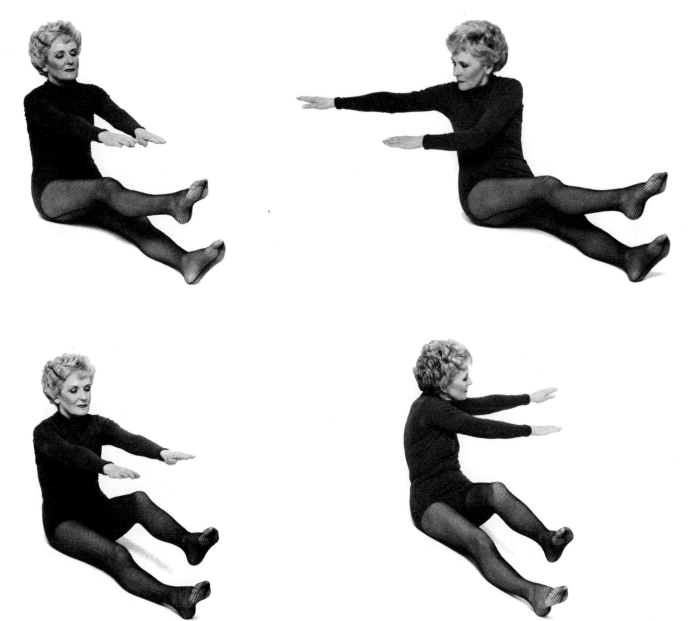

2. Now raise the left leg slightly.

3. Twist body and arms to the left side as far as you can. Twist 3 times.

Alternating right and left legs, do exercise 20 times.

ABDOMEN/3

Starting Position: Sit on the floor with your back pressed against the wall. Extend legs and bend knees just far enough to bring the soles of your feet together. Throughout this exercise, keep the small of your back pressed against the wall by firmly pulling your stomach in.

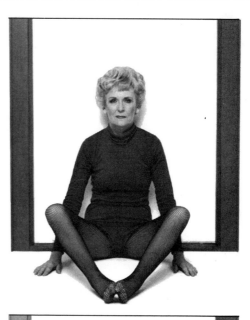

Movements:

1. Take a deep breath as you raise both arms above your head, bringing your elbows as close to the wall as possible.

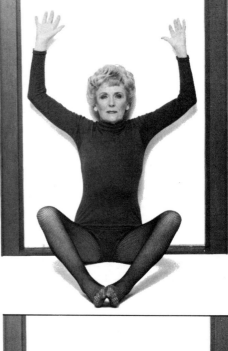

2. Bring arms and shoulders forward and touch your toes. Expel the air from your lungs as you come forward.

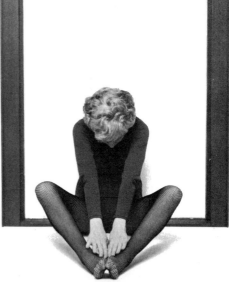

Do exercise 10 times.

Starting Position: Stand with feet comfortably apart.

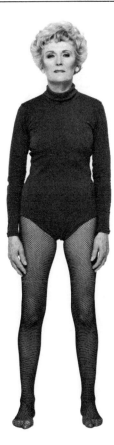

Movements:

1. Bend your knees and bring the pelvic region forward as far as you can.

2. Straighten the knees and slowly move the pelvic region back until your rump sticks out and you are standing "sway-backed."

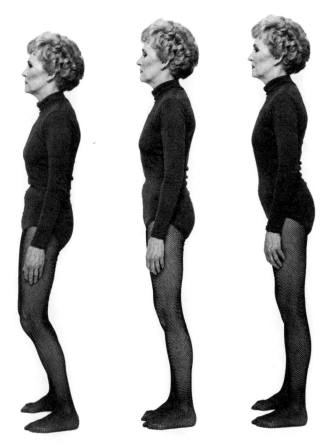

Do exercise 10 times.

ABDOMEN/5

Starting Position: Stand with feet approximately 16 inches apart and bend your knees. Pull your stomach in as tightly as you can.

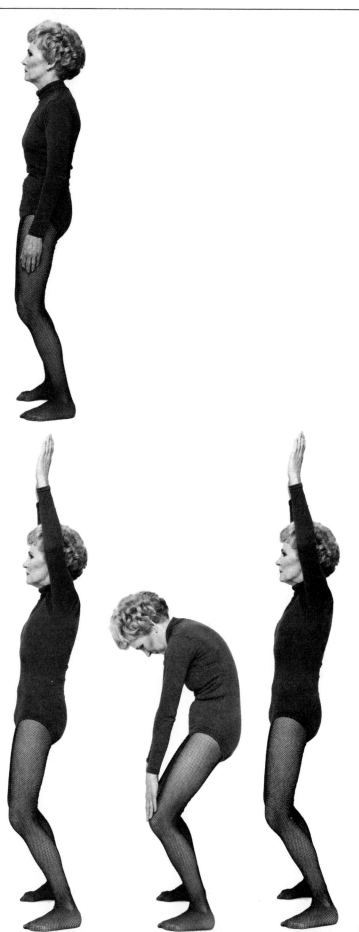

Movements:

1. Stretch arms up over your head.

2. Keep pulling your stomach in as you bring your hands to your bent knees.

3. Again, raise arms up over your head.

Do exercise 10 times.

Starting Position: Stand with hands clasped behind your neck.

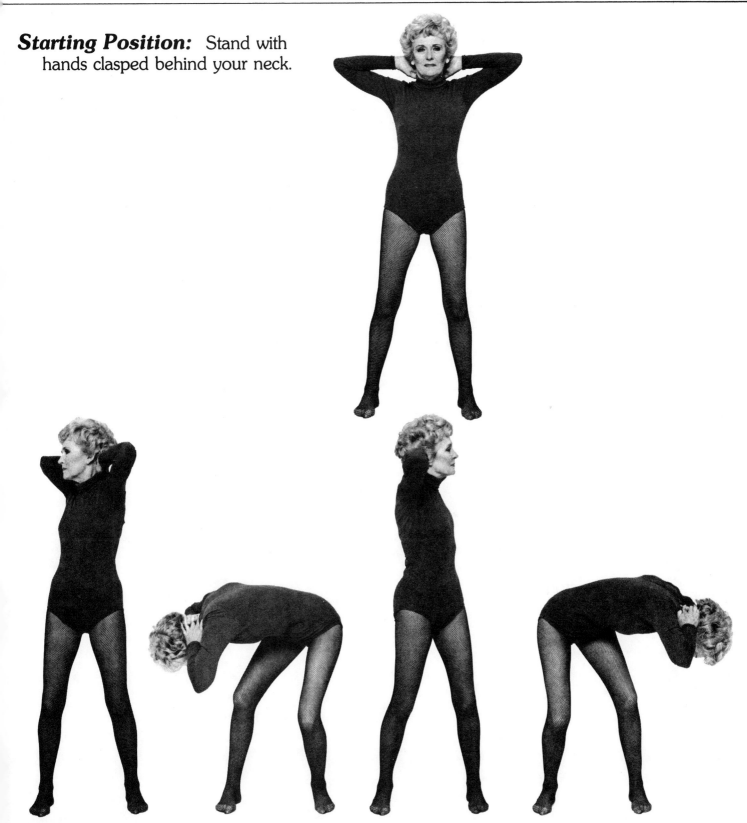

Movements:

1. Turn body to the right. Hold the turn, and bow by bending at the waist.

2. Bring body to an upright position and turn to the left. Bow.

Do exercise 10 times (5 times on each side).

ABDOMEN/7

Starting Position: Stand about 3 feet from a table. Bend at the waist, adjusting the position so that your fingertips are about 12 inches from the edge of the table.

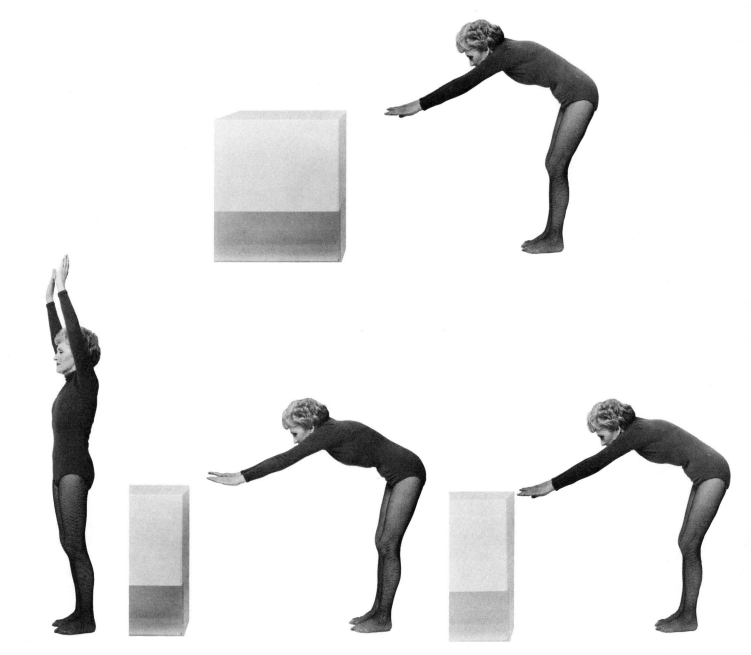

Movements:

1. Straighten your body. Bring arms up over your head.

2. Raise your chest.

3. Bend at the waist again. Stretch torso toward table as if trying to touch it with your outstretched fingers. Pull your stomach in as you stretch.

Do exercise 10 times.

Starting Position: Stand about a foot away from a table, with your hands pressing down on the tabletop and your elbows locked in a straight position.

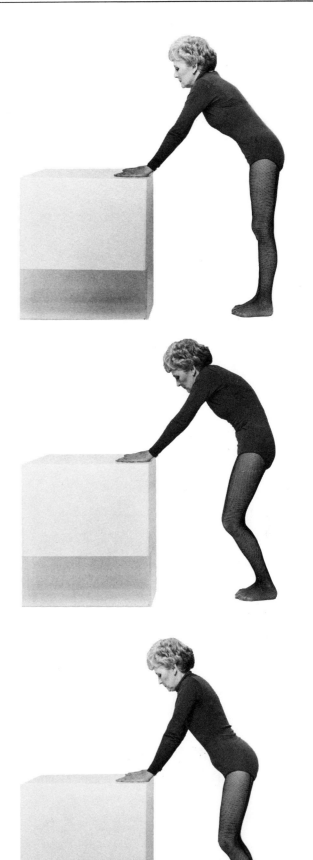

Movements:

1. Bend knees and pull stomach in. Keep it pulled in and lift it up.

2. Hold the stomach pulled in and up for a count of about 5.

3. At the count of 5 relax the stomach muscles and literally let your abdomen "drop."

Do exercise 10 times.

ANKLES AND ARCHES

The muscles and tendons of the ankles and arches are used for extension, flexion, inversion and eversion, and are capable of minute adjustments that help to keep the body in balance. These muscles and tendons work in conjunction with those of the lower leg. The ankle joint is sprained more frequently than any other joint in the body, and people's most common complaint is aching feet. The way one walks or stands and the shoes one wears affect the condition of the ankles, feet and toes.

In order to strengthen the muscles which permit more running, standing or walking without pain, it is necessary to exercise those muscles which are rarely used in today's normal activities.

The exercises in this section will be more beneficial if they are done in bare feet.

ANKLES AND ARCHES/1

Starting Position: Sit with the left leg crossed over the right knee. Press the thumb of your right hand on the metatarsal arch.

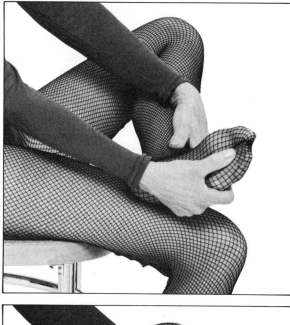

Movements:

1. Bend your toes down.

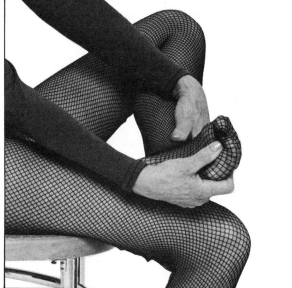

2. Bend your toes up.

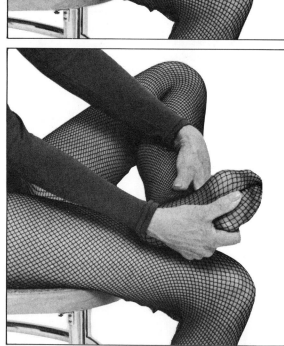

Do these movements 20 times.
Reverse the position of your legs and do exercise 20 times with the other foot.

Starting Position: Sit on a chair with feet parallel to each other and flat on the floor.

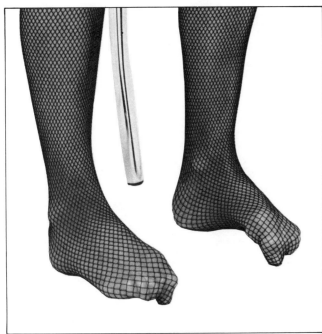

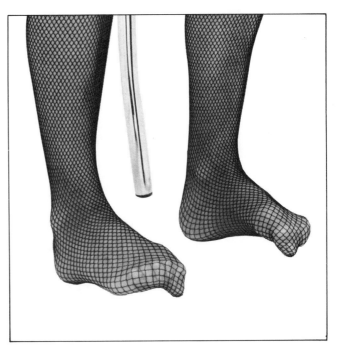

Movements:

1. Squeeze your toes together and keep them that way.

2. Keeping heels on the floor, lift toes up.

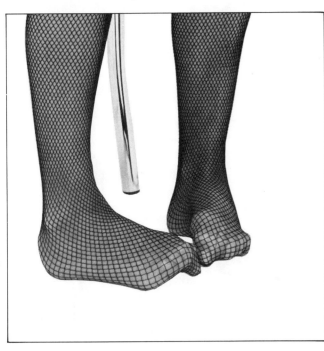

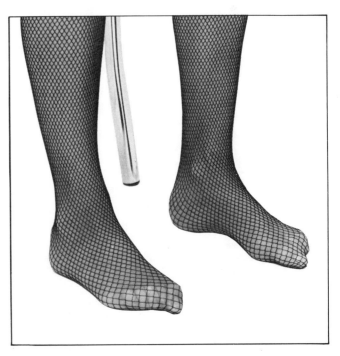

3. In this raised position, turn your feet inward until the toes touch.

4. Return feet to starting position.

Do exercise 10 times.

ANKLES AND ARCHES/3

Starting Position: Sit on the edge of a chair with heels lifted and the weight of your feet resting on curled-up toes.

Movements:

1. Straighten the curled toes, stretching them out.

2. Curl them again.

Do movements 20 times.

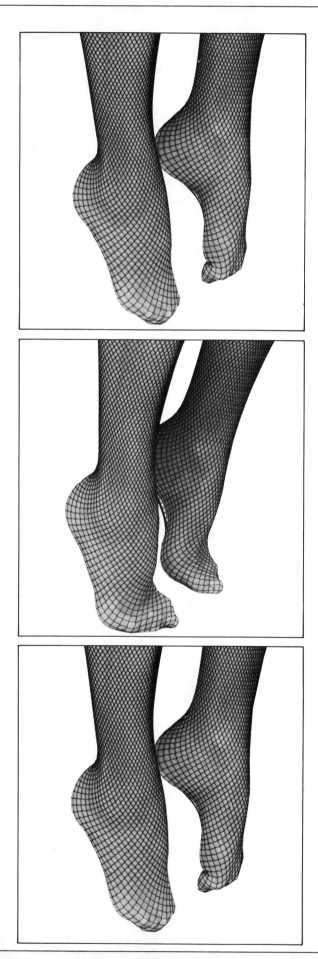

Starting Position: Stand with feet flat on the floor, about 6 inches apart and parallel to each other.

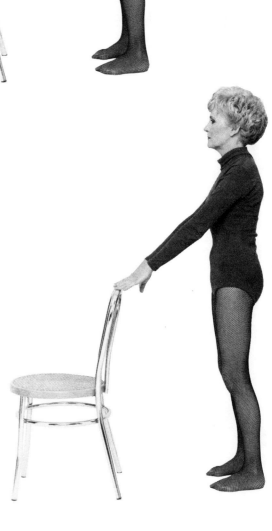

Movements:

1. Raise heels and stand on your toes.

2. Return heels to the floor.

Do movements 20 times.

Starting Position: Stand with your back leaning against a wall.

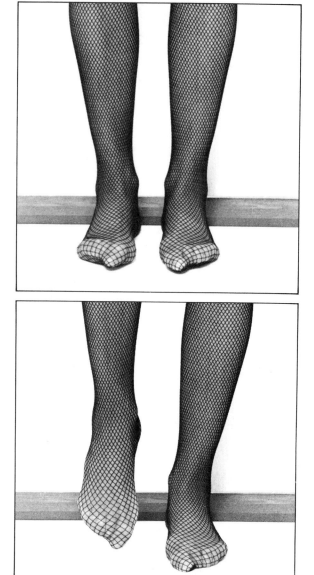

Movements:

1. Raise the right foot.

2. Point your toes toward the floor and hold them for a few seconds in that position.

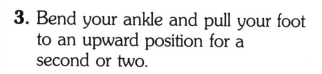

3. Bend your ankle and pull your foot to an upward position for a second or two.

4. Relax.

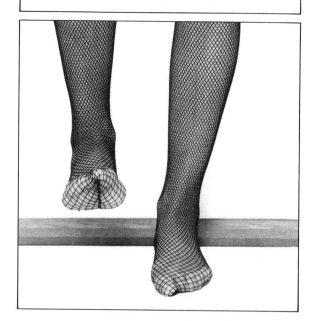

Do upward and downward movements 10 times slowly, then 10 times quickly. Change legs and repeat exercise with left foot lifted.

Starting Position: Stand with your back against a wall. Place the right foot slightly in front of the left.

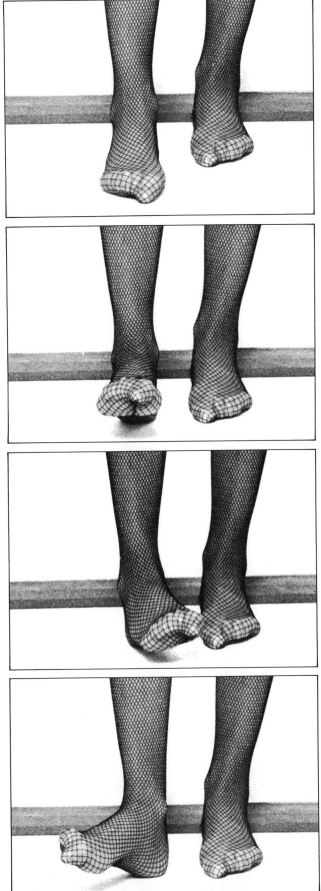

Movements:

1. Raise the forepart of the right foot, resting its weight on the heel.

2. With the foot resting on the heel, turn the foot inward and hold it in that position for a second or two.

3. Turn the foot outward and hold it in that position for a second or two.

Do this inward-outward movement 20 times. Repeat exercise with the left foot extended.

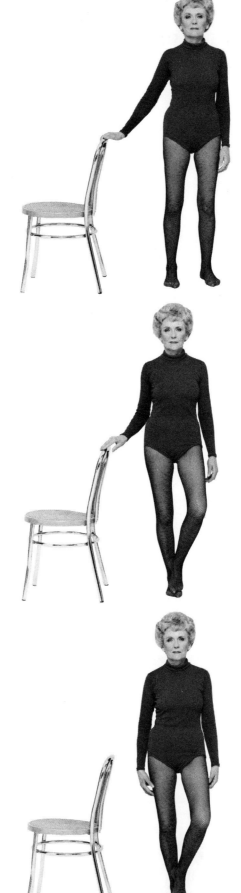

Starting Position: Stand with your hand resting on the back of a chair for balance.

Movements:

1. Place the left foot on top of the right foot.

2. Find a fixed point on the wall and stare at it.

3. Take your hand away from the chair.

4. Stand in this position as long as you can.

Repeat exercise with right foot on top of left foot.

This exercise is especially good for tennis players and joggers, who often suffer from painful pulls of the Achilles tendon. This tendon shortens from lack of use, and needs to be lengthened before one participates in active sports.

Starting Position: Stand with your back to a wall, with the balls of the feet resting on a book that is at least 2 inches thick.

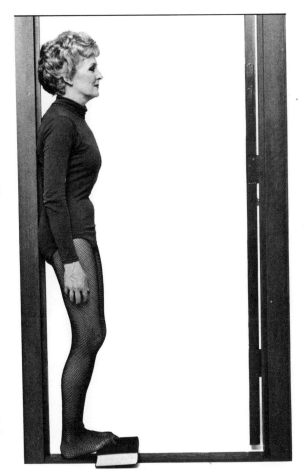

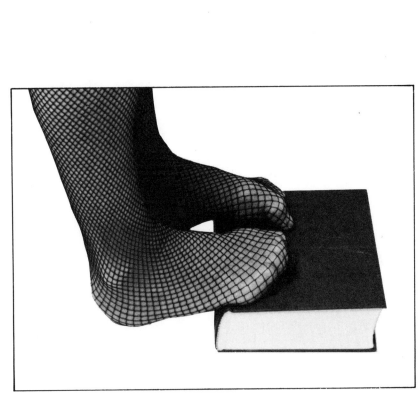

Movements:
Rest heels on floor. Without lifting them, roll your weight to the outside of your feet. Hold the feet in that position as long as you can. Relax.

Do this exercise at least 20 times daily.

ARMS

The biceps of the upper arm are responsible for bending the elbow; the triceps are used for returning the arm to a straightened position. These two muscles work in concert with the muscles in the forearm and hand and those of the shoulder joint to bring other movements to the arms: rotation, abduction, aduction, flexion and extension.

When the hands and wrists are moved for normal tasks, the forearm muscles are being exercised. The upper-arm muscles come into play for larger chores such as reaching, lifting, pushing and carrying weight.

Depending, therefore, on your occupation or daily habits, you may find the muscles of the upper arms beginning to lose their tone and becoming frankly flabby.

Help is at hand with the following exercises. While all arm muscles will come into play, these are particularly designed to concentrate on working the muscles of the upper arms.

ARMS/1

Starting Position: Standing or sitting, extend arms to the sides at shoulder level, with palms turned up.

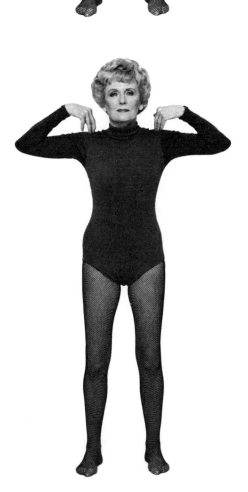

Movements:

1. Touch tips of fingers to tops of shoulders.

2. Straighten arms to starting position.

Do exercise 25 times.

Starting Position: Stand with elbows bent and press arms against your ears, with palms of your hands resting on the center upper back.

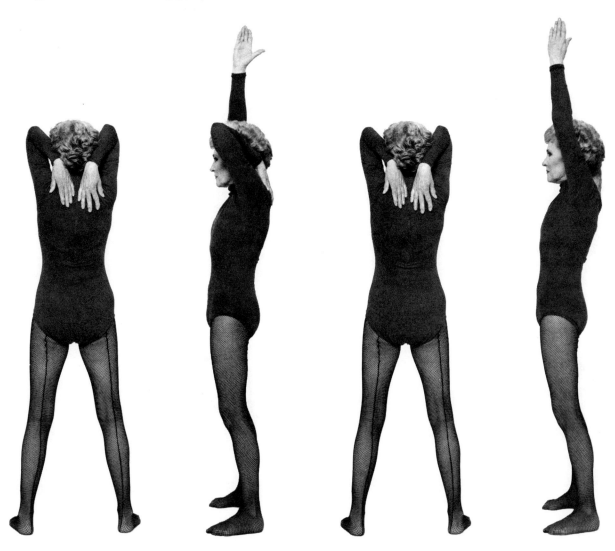

Movements:

1. Keeping one arm pressed against your head, raise the other arm and point it toward the ceiling.

2. Return arm to starting position.

Repeat movements with the other arm.

Do movements 40 times (20 times with each arm).

ARMS/3

Starting Position: Stand with arms raised at shoulder level in front of you, with palms down.

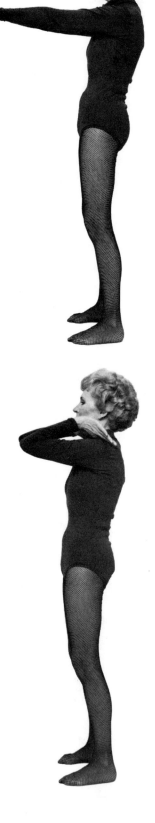

Movements:

1. Bend elbows and bring the backs of the hands up to touch your shoulders.

2. Bring arms back to starting position.

Do exercise 25 times.

Starting Position: Stand with feet apart and arms raised in front of you at shoulder level.

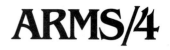

Movements:

1. Clench your hands.

2. Bring both arms simultaneously down to the sides of the body.

3. Raise arms in back of the body as far up as you can. Release the fists and bring arms back up to starting position.

Do exercise 25 times.

ARMS/5

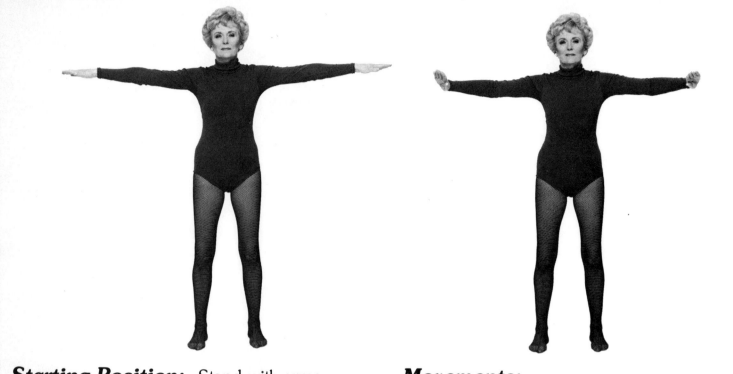

Starting Position: Stand with arms extended to the side at shoulder level.

Movements:
1. Turn the wrists inward—until they will not go any farther.

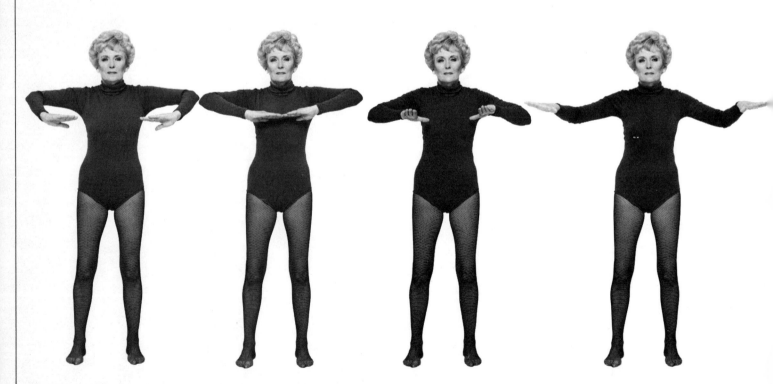

2. Now keep turning them until the elbows actually bend as a result of moving the wrists inward toward your chest.

Do exercise 20 times.

3. Slowly straighten the wrists and push them back in the other direction, which will straighten your elbows.

Starting Position: Stand with feet parallel to each other. Keep elbows as straight as possible and place your palms on your buttocks.

Movements:

1. Keeping the left hand on your buttock, raise the right hand and bring it down to slap the buttock 10 times.

2. Keeping the right hand on your buttock, raise the left hand and bring it down to slap the buttock 10 times.

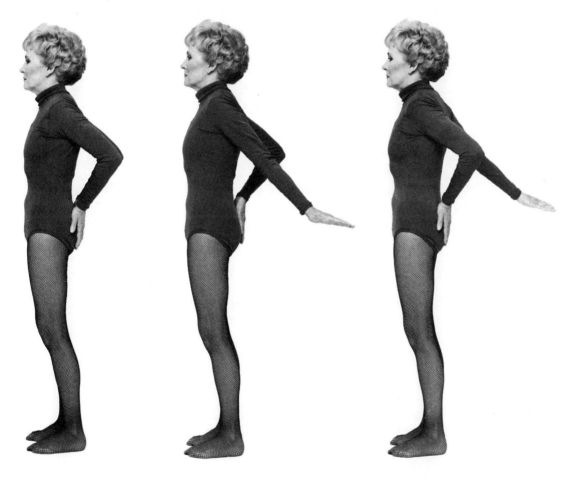

Alternate the slaps—first with the right hand and then with the left—another 10 times.

Starting Position: Stand with elbows bent at shoulder level and hands in front of your chest, palms down and fingertips touching.

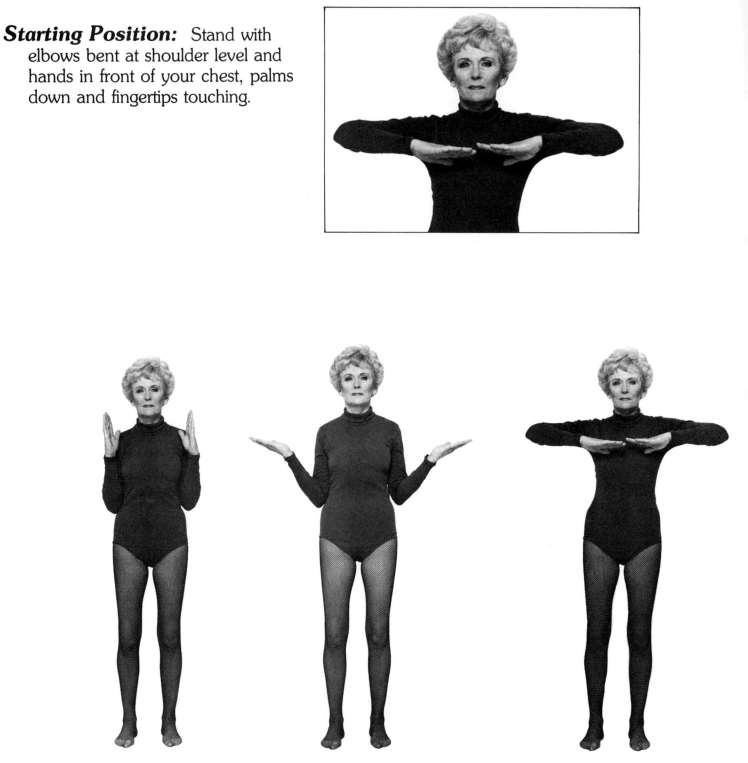

Movements:

1. Bring arms down—with elbows still bent—and pull elbows in close to your body.

2. Keeping elbows pressed close to the body, move the forearms so that your palms face up. Return arms to starting position.

Do exercise 20 times.

Starting Position: Extend arms in front of you, with the backs of the hands touching each other.

Movements:

1. Slowly separate hands, bringing your arms out to the side at shoulder level.

2. Bend elbows and bring arms and hands back to starting position, thus making a circle with each arm, as in the breast stroke.

Make 25 circles.

BOSOM AND CHEST

The muscles of the chest are called the pectorals. It is these muscles which work together with those of the arms, shoulders and back, and which keep the bosoms lifted. If the muscles lose their tone, the bosoms sag.

The bosom size cannot be enlarged through exercise, though chest measurements can be increased by using heavy weights and doing other strenuous calisthenics. The exercises in this section are based on natural movements designed to lift the bosom and firm the chest muscles rather than to increase chest measurements.

BOSOM AND CHEST/1

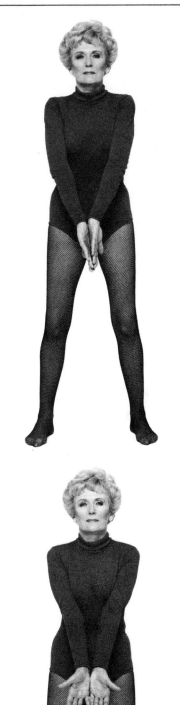

Starting Position: Stand with arms down in front of your body, backs of hands touching. Keep arms and shoulders in this forward position throughout the exercise.

Movements:

1. Twist arms until your palms face forward and the little fingers touch each other.

2. Twist arms back to starting postion.

Do these twists 20 times.

Starting Position: Stand with feet planted firmly on the floor. Put hands behind your back and clasp the fingers of the right hand with your left hand.

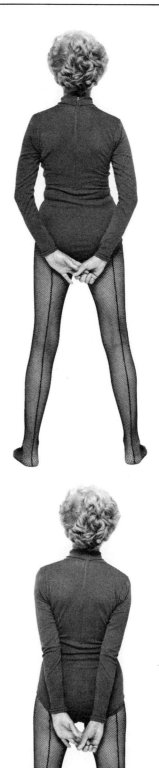

Movements:

1. Lift your chest and pull hands down toward the floor. Then lift the chest even higher.

2. Relax.

Do exercise 15 times.

BOSOM AND CHEST/3

Starting Position: Stand with feet planted firmly on the floor. Stretch arms out to the side at shoulder level, with palms facing forward.

Movements:

1. Twist the left arm and bring it across the body to touch back of hand to the extended right forearm. (Keep the elbows of both arms as straight as possible.)

2. Return the left arm to its starting position.

Do this exercise 10 times with the left arm. Then do the same movements with the right arm, crossing the body 10 times.

Starting Position: Stand with feet planted firmly on the floor. Hold arms at shoulder level, with elbows bent.

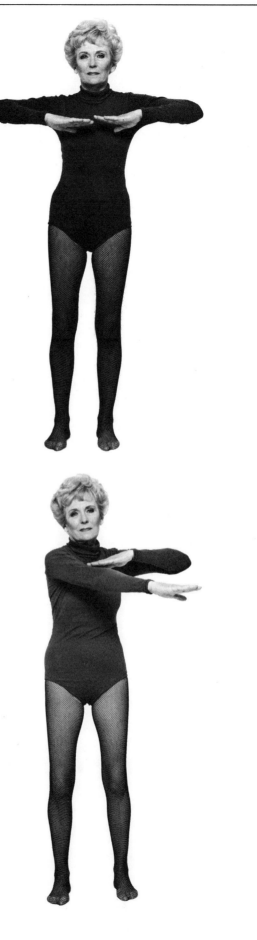

Movements:

1. Straighten the right arm and bring it across your body.

2. Bring arm back to its starting position.

Do this exercise 20 times with the right arm, then 20 times with the left arm.

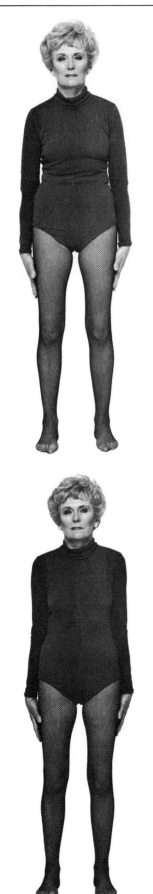

Starting Position: Stand with arms at your sides, pressing the fingertips to the thighs as far down on your legs as you can reach.

Movements:

1. Press the insides of your arms against the sides of the body.

2. Hold arms against your sides for a second or two and then relax them.

Do these movements 10 times.

Starting Position: Stand with feet apart, arms extended to the side at shoulder level and palms facing down.

Movements:

1. Keep elbows straight by tensing the arms, then bring both arms down to your sides.

2. Keeping arms tense, return them to shoulder level.

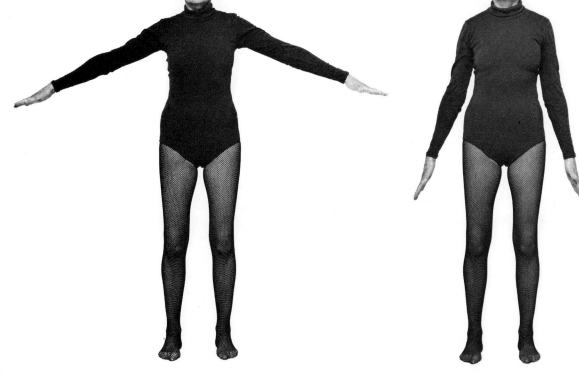

Do this "flying" with tensed-arm motion 20 times.

BOSOM AND CHEST/7

Starting Position: Stand with arms at your sides.

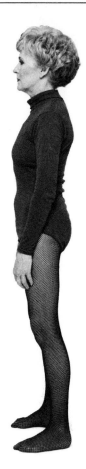

Movements:

1. Press arms against the body and lift the chest as high as you can without lifting your shoulders.

2. Breathe in.

3. Relax the chest and expel the breath.

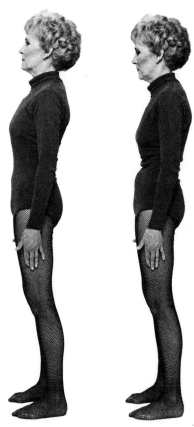

Do exercise 10 times.

Starting Position: Stand with arms extended to the side, palms facing up.

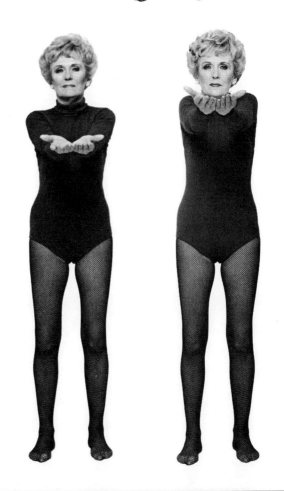

Movements:

1. Swing arms forward. Try (you can't) to bring the insides of your elbows together.

2. Pull your shoulders up to your ears. Spread arms to starting position.

3. Roll your shoulders back and down to the starting postion.

Do exercise 10 times.

BUTTOCKS AND HIPS

Bumps and lumps and sags and flab are the words generally used to describe what is wrong with the hip-and-buttock area of the body. Unless one is active, these unattractive features are very easy to come by. Those who have to sit a great deal find their hips just "naturally" spread. The way one sits can make some difference (for instance, sitting forward in a chair with the spine straight helps— see "Posture"), but one also needs to concentrate specifically on toning the muscles of the hips and buttocks in order to get the best results.

The muscles which bring tone and shape to the buttock-and-hip area are those which raise the hips and move the thighs backward, forward, outward and inward. These are the movements we are concerned with in the following exercises.

BUTTOCKS AND HIPS/1

Starting Position: Stand with right hand resting on the back of a chair. Bend the left knee and put your foot behind you.

Movements:

1. Lift the left hip in an upward direction.

2. Keeping knee bent, return hip to natural position.

Raise and lower hip in this manner 10 times.

Turn, and using left hand for support, do exercise 10 times, raising right hip.

Starting Position: Stand with right hand resting on the back of a chair or table for support. Put your weight on the right foot. Bend the left knee and raise its foot and leg behind you.

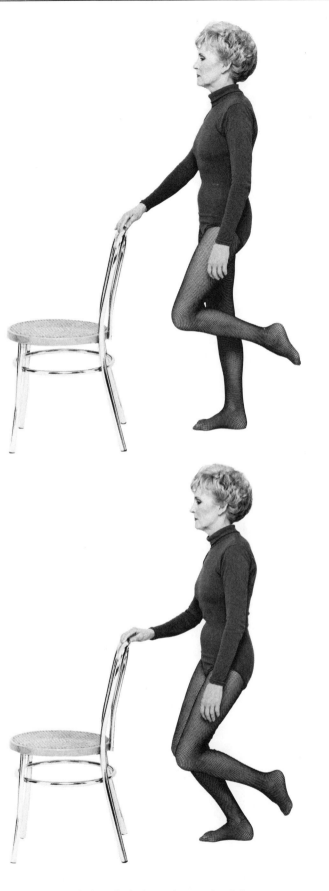

Movements:

1. Bend the knee of the leg supporting your weight (the right knee) as slowly as you can.

2. Bend and straighten the right knee slowly and rhythmically 8 times.

Repeat exercise, bending and straightening the knee of the left leg (as it holds the body's weight), 8 times.

BUTTOCKS AND HIPS/3

Starting Position: You will need a chair or table to lean on. Bend your body at the waist and put elbows and forearms on the table or chair. Keep knees straight and put left foot directly behind you, resting its weight on the toes.

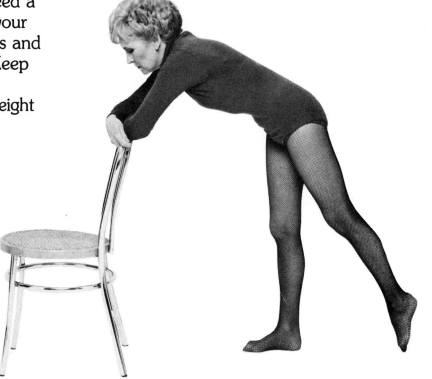

Movements:
(Do this exercise in SLOW motion.)

1. Raise the left leg to hip level, and hold it there for the count of 5.

2. Return the left leg to its starting position as slowly as you can.

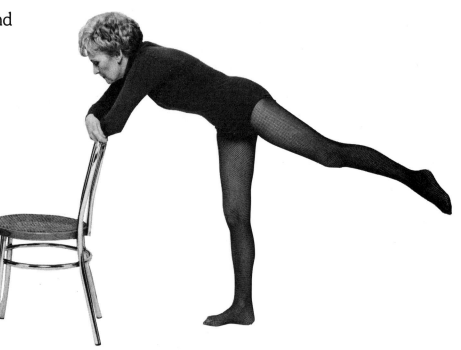

Do exercise 8 times.

Repeat exercise with right leg.

Starting Position: Stand with right hand resting on the back of a chair. Bend left knee and raise leg.

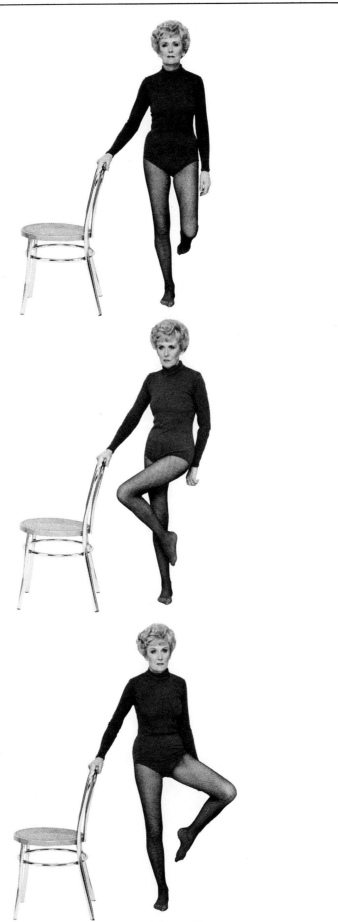

Movements:

1. Swing bent knee in toward the chair.

2. Swing it out, away from the chair.

Swing leg in and out 10 times.

SWING IT SLOWLY!

Repeat exercise with other leg.

BUTTOCKS AND HIPS/5

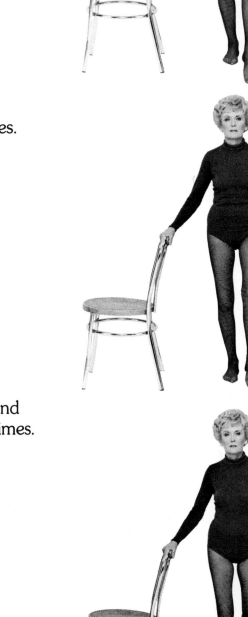

Starting Position: Stand next to a chair, with right hand resting on it. Move the left leg forward so that just the tips of its toes rest on the floor.

Movements:

1. Lift toes slightly off the floor 20 times.

2. Now move the left leg directly behind you, and again lift toes slightly 15 times.

Repeat exercise with the other leg.

Starting Position: Stand with right hand resting on the back of a chair. Bring left leg out to the side, foot raised so that toes only are touching the floor.

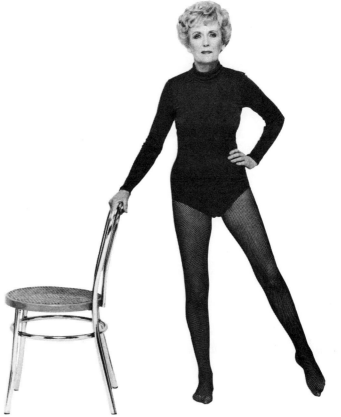

Movements:

1. Keeping toes on the floor, move foot directly behind the right leg.

2. Still keeping toes on the floor, return leg to its starting position.

Do exercise 10 times.

Turn and do exercise with other leg.

BUTTOCKS AND HIPS/7

Starting Position: Stand with right hand resting on the back of a chair. Bend left knee and bring leg in back of you. The foot should be about 10 inches from the floor.

Movements:

1. With knee bent, push the thigh forward and hold it in this forward position for a count of 5.

2. Push the thigh back behind your body as far as you can and hold it for a count of 5.

(Remember not to straighten the knee in this exercise so that you will force the muscles in the thigh and buttock area to do all the work.)

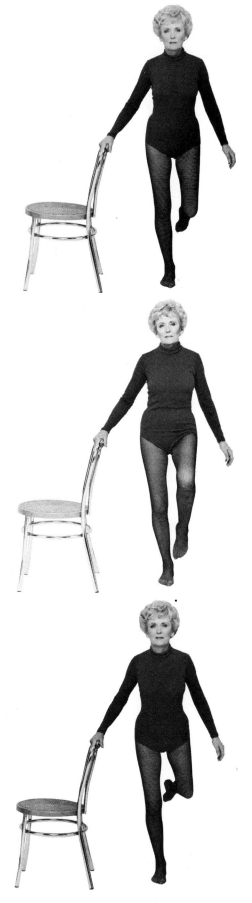

Do exercise 10 times with left knee bent, then 10 times with right knee bent.

Starting Position: Bend your body at the waist and lean your elbows and forearms on a chair back or table.

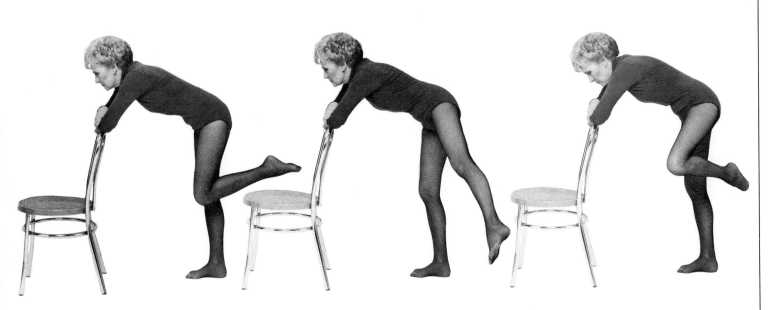

Movements:

1. Bend the left knee and bring foot up behind you at thigh level.

2. Straighten the knee and extend the leg to the side. Hold it there for a count of 2.

3. Slowly bend the knee and bring it back alongside the right knee.

Do exercise 10 times; then do it 10 more times with the other leg.

CALVES

The muscles of the calves work together with those of the ankle, feet and thigh. The Achilles tendon joins the calf to the heel bone. The calf muscles are partially responsible for balancing the body on the foot, bringing the thighs to the kneeling position, raising the heel from the floor and extending the foot.

Even though these calf muscles come into constant use when one walks, runs, dances and jumps, they are rarely used to their fullest capacity. The Achilles tendon is almost always foreshortened in those who constantly wear high heels and otherwise fail to stretch it to its fullest length. The exercises in this section are designed to stretch this tendon and to bring strength to the potentially powerful calf muscles, which can become extremely weakened by lack of use. If further work is needed, turn to "Ankles and Arches."

Note: All exercises in this section should be done in bare feet.

CALVES/1

Starting Position: Sit on a chair with feet flat on the floor.

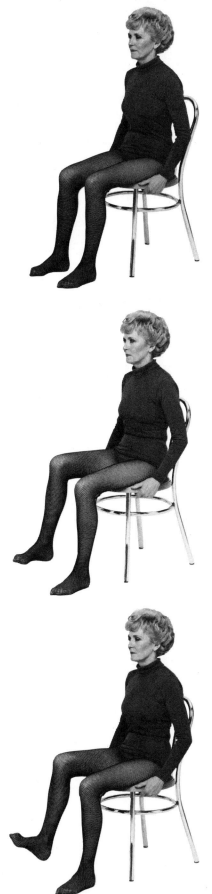

Movements:

1. Keeping the knee bent, lift the right foot off the floor.

2. Holding the knee and leg in this lifted position, turn the foot upward.

3. Still holding the knee, leg and foot lifted, turn only the foot outward. Hold this position for a few seconds before returning to starting position.

Do exercise 5 times. Then repeat it with the other leg.

Starting Position: Stand with the left hand resting on the back of a chair, heels touching and toes pointed away from each other.

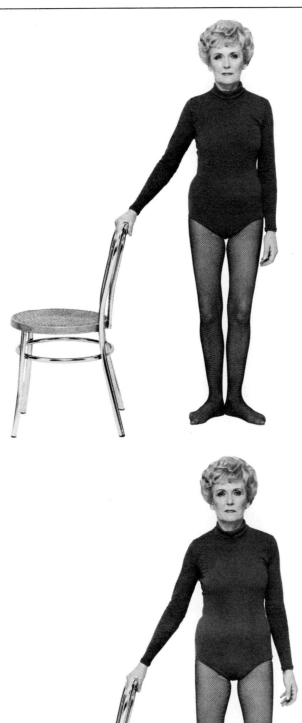

Movements:

1. Lift heels from the floor and stand on your toes.

2. Return heels to the floor.

Do exercise 20 times.

CALVES/3

Starting Position: Stand with feet firmly planted on the floor, about 12 inches apart and parallel to each other.

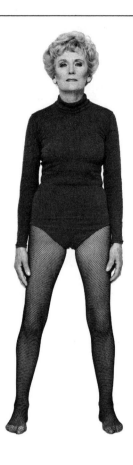

Movements:

1. Keeping your back upright, bend your knees as deeply as possible without lifting your heels from the floor. Be conscious of letting the calves of the legs hold the weight of your body.

2. Hold the calves in this stretched position. Then, when you begin to feel the strain, bounce 3 or 4 times to stretch the calf muscles even more.

3. Straighten the knees and relax.

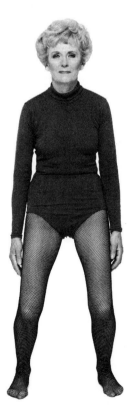

Do exercise 5 times.

Starting Position: Stand with the right hand resting on the back of a chair. Place the bottom of your left foot against your ankle, resting the weight of the foot on the tips of the toes.

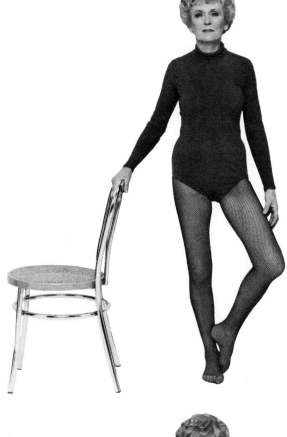

Movements:

1. Move your heel away from your leg.

2. Return heel to your leg.

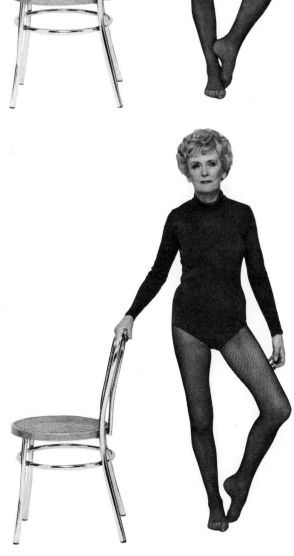

Do exercise 10 times with each leg.

CALVES/5

Starting Position: Stand with feet wide apart and turned outward.

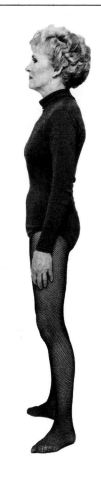

Movements:

1. Keeping the feet firmly on the floor, bend knees and body and bring hands down to the floor.

2. Stay in this position for a count of 5.

3. Raise to starting position without moving your feet.

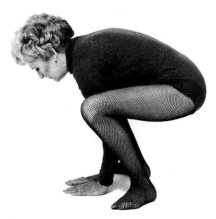

Bend over and stand up 10 times.

Starting Position: Stand with the right hand resting on the back of a chair. Turn your toes inward to an exaggerated "pigeon-toed" position.

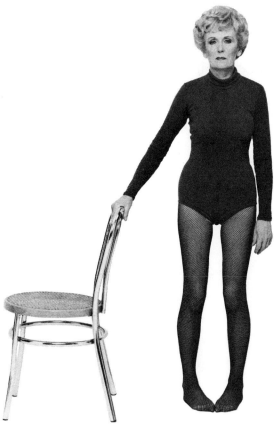

Movements:

1. Keeping the feet "pigeon-toed," roll your weight to the outside of the foot.

2. Return feet to starting position.

Do exercise 10 times.

CALVES/7

Starting Position: Stand and place your hands on a wall at shoulder level, with elbows locked in a straight position. Move legs back from the wall as far as you can and still keep heels on the floor; lock your knees.

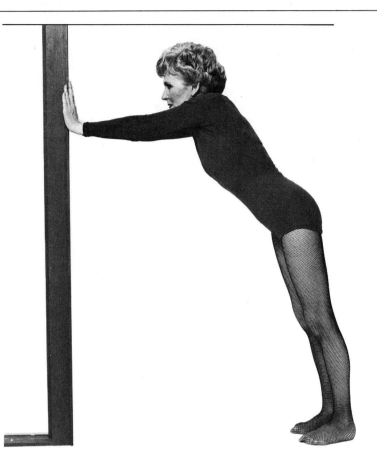

Movements:

(The movement is slight but effective.)

1. With knees and elbows locked, lean body slightly in toward wall until you feel a great stretch in the calf muscles.

2. Hold the "lean" for the count of 10 (or longer, if you can).

3. Relax for a few seconds.

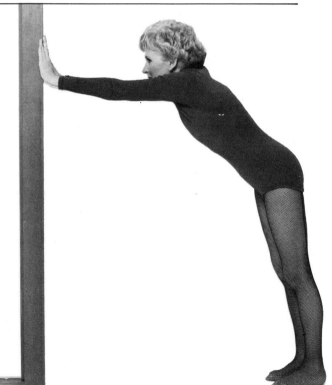

Do exercise 5 times.

JUMPING is one of the quick ways of bringing calf muscles into tone—and curiously, while jumping, one automatically exercises the heart muscle. The obvious way to do this is, of course, with a jump rope. But that would require more space (and soundproofing) than most modern buildings have; however, jumping with an "imaginary" rope doesn't, and the exercise is the same. The following can be done with or without a rope.

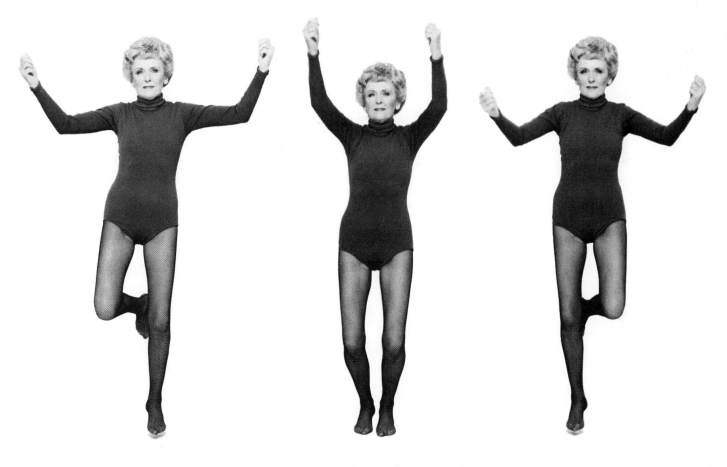

Jump first on one foot, then on the other.

Jump with both feet at same time.

Jump one-legged.

Do all the jumps you did as a child.

Quit when you get tired.

FACE

The exercises in this section are taken from my book Miss Craig's Face-Saving Exercises, which has a six-day plan to improve sagging facial muscles. These muscles—like those of the rest of the body —have a natural job to do. I developed these natural movements into a series of exercises which help to bring tone to the muscles and to the skin of the face. The ones I have selected for inclusion here do not involve all the facial muscles, but only those that are concerned with the areas which my private clients seem to need the most (the headings on each of the eight exercises indicate these particular areas).

Once the movements have been learned, it is advisable to run through them on a regular, if not daily, basis for the best results—that is, to bring the muscles of the face to tone and to help to keep them in that condition.

"Double chins" can be caused by excessive weight, improper head carriage and sitting and standing postures. If additional toning is needed for the double-chin area, turn to the "Posture" and "Neck" sections.

FACE/1

To Help Alleviate Vertical Frown Lines

Starting Position: Face mirror squarely, with eyes open.

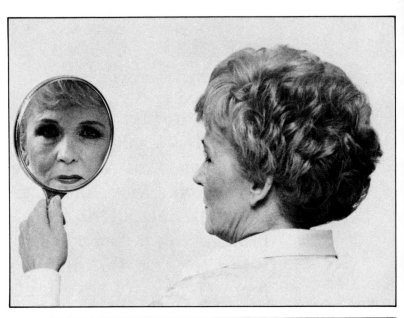

Movements:

1. Pull your eyebrows way down over your eyes. In other words, really frown. Frown so hard that it will feel as though you were trying to get your eyebrows to meet each other. Think "frown" as you frown.

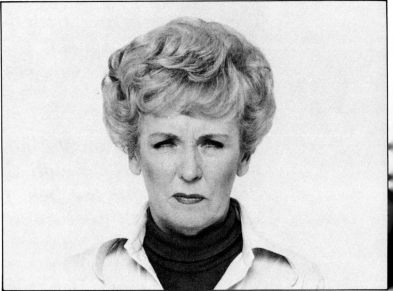

2. Then lift your eyebrows as high—and open your eyes as wide—as you can.

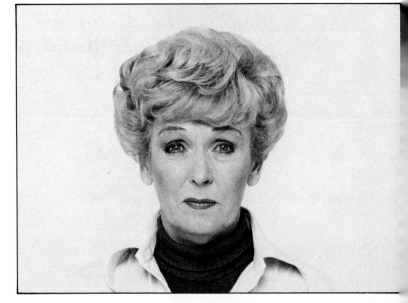

Do exercise 8 times, counting each time you frown.

To Tone Eyelid Area

Starting Position: Close your eyes into a tight squeeze.

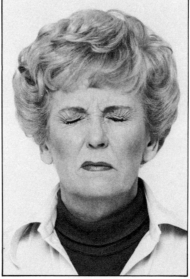

Movements:

1. Then think of squeezing your eyes even more tightly closed—and do it. Let the cheek muscles help you.

2. Now, think of releasing the squeeze— and do it.

DO IT SLOWLY.

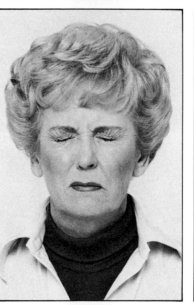
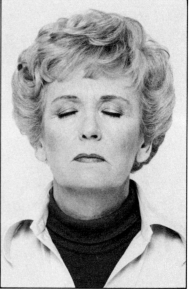

3. Lift the eyebrows and stretch the upper lids as wide as you can over your closed eyes. Really stretch those eyelids.

4. Slowly release the stretch.

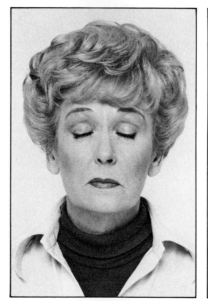
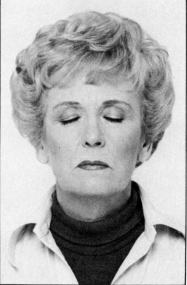

Do exercise 8 times, counting each time you squeeze eyes closed.

FACE/3

To Tone Under-Eye Area

Starting Position: Stand close to a mirror. Raise your eyebrows and lift upper lids until you see the whites of your eyes above the iris.

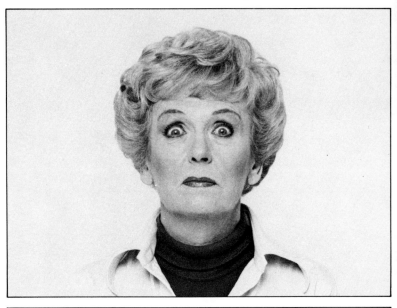

Movements:

1. Slowly begin to bring the upper and lower lids together until you appear slit-eyed. Think about both lids resisting each other as you bring them together.

   (To do this properly, you will need to concentrate. The upper lids should not move down at a faster rate than the lower lids move up.)

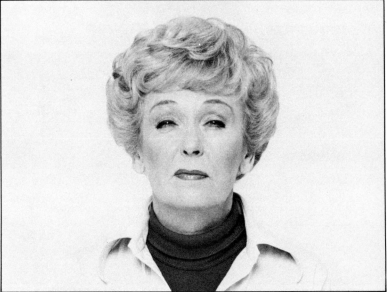

2. Now slowly open your eyes, again thinking of resisting as you concentrate on moving the upper and lower lids apart at the same slow pace.

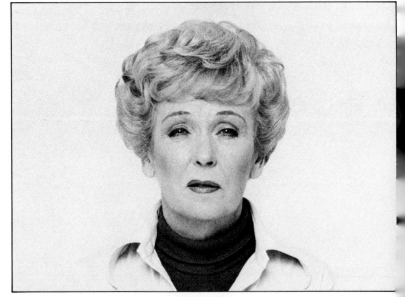

Do exercise 8 times, counting each time lids are brought together.

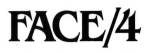

To Tone and Firm Cheek Area

Starting Position: Get close to a mirror. Raise your eyebrows. Make a crooked grin with the right side of your mouth. Hold that position throughout exercise.

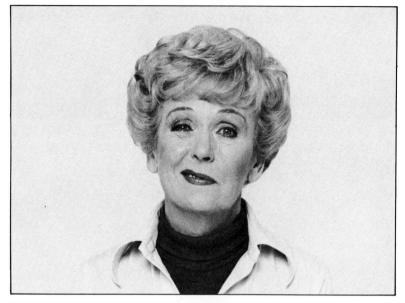

Movements:

1. Place right index finger on cheek below outer corner of right eye. Your finger is now resting on the muscle to be exercised.

2. Think about this muscle and use it to slowly push the lower lid of your right eye closed. Hold. Then slowly return to normal position.

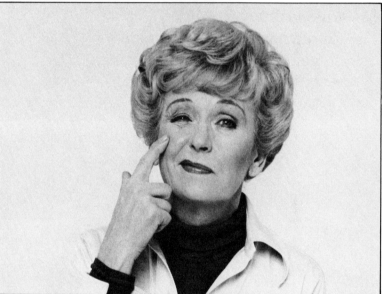

3. Repeat all the above movements with left eye.

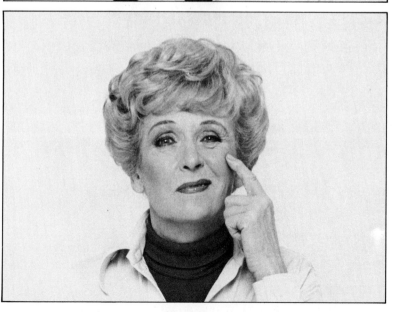

Do exercise 8 times, counting each time you close right eye.

FACE/5

To Alleviate Jowls and Firm the Throat Area

Starting Position: Hold your head upright throughout exercise, with chin tilted up slightly and lips firmly closed.

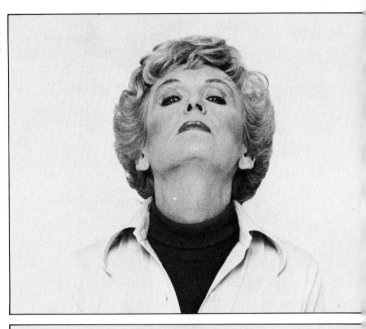

Movements:

1. Slowly separate lower teeth from upper teeth, getting as much distance between them as you can without letting lips part.

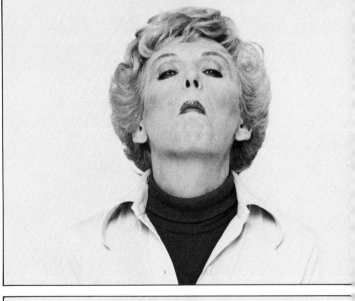

2. Slowly return teeth to normal position, to conclude one exaggerated "chewing" motion.

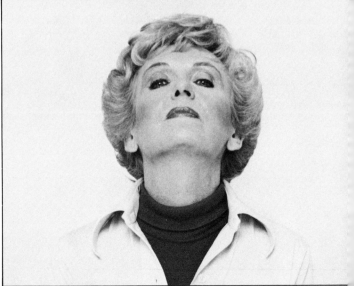

Do exercise 20 times, counting each time you separate teeth.

To Tone the Smile Area
at the Corners of the Mouth

Starting Position: Smile with your lips together, turning corners of mouth in an upward direction.

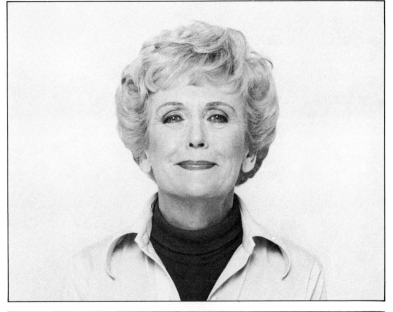

Movements:

1. Keep smiling upward and separate your iips to make a "toothless" upward smile. In other words, cover your teeth with your lips.

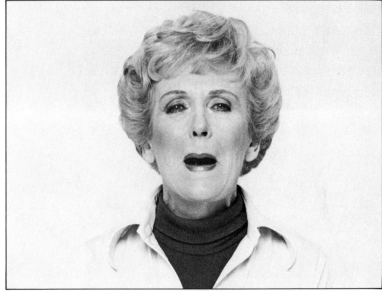

2. Now, still keeping your teeth covered, slowly bring your mouth to an "O" shape.

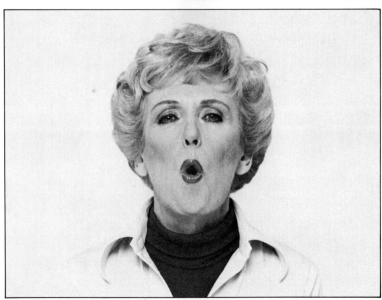

Do exercise 8 times, counting each time you smile.

FACE/7

To Tone Furrow Area from Mouth Corners to Chin

Starting Position: Lift lower lip up to a slight "pout" position.

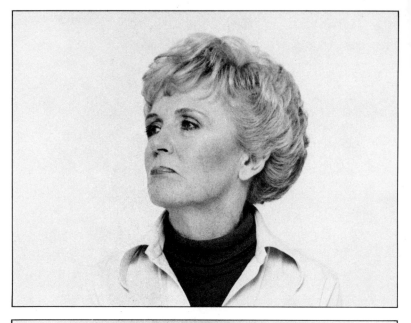

Movements:

1. Keep pout as much as you can and pucker the lower lip, as if you were trying to make its two corners meet in the center of the mouth.

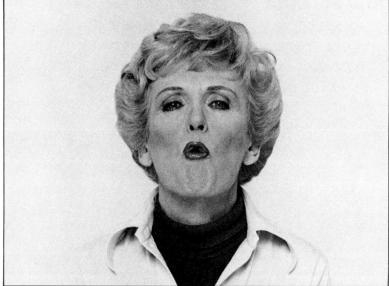

2. Slowly release pucker . . .
. . . to return mouth to natural position.

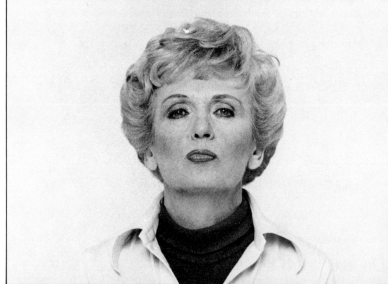

Do exercise 8 times, counting each time you pucker lower lip.

To Help Lesson Furrows from Mouth Corners to Chin

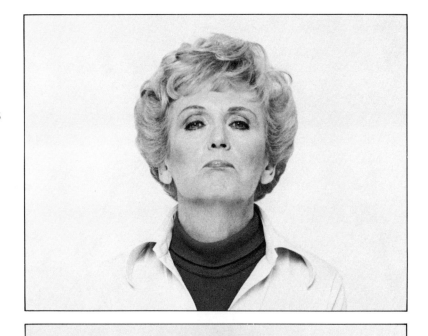

Starting Position: Bring your lips to a pursed postion.

Movements:

1. Use the muscle at the tip of your chin to push "pursed" lips upward. When lips are pushed up as far as they will go . . .

2. . . . hold the upward tension with your chin and pull the corners of your mouth downward. Hold downward contraction for the count of 5.

3. Then slowly return lips to horizontal position.

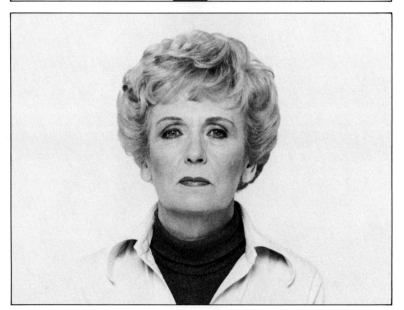

Do exercise 8 times, counting each time you push lips upward.

FINGERS

The muscles of the fingers and hand work in concert with those of the wrist and forearm. The fingers have many joints for their muscles to move, but rarely, in everyday life, do we move all of them—unless an occupation or hobby demands it. This accounts for the fact that as one grows older, the hands lose their strength and dexterity.

The muscles of the hand extend and flex the fingers, move them toward and away from one another, and also rotate them at the knuckles.

Exercises help to keep the joints of the hands from becoming stiff. If additional toning is needed, turn to the "Wrists" section.

FINGERS/1

Starting Position: Hold your
hands in front of your chest.

Movements:

1. Make tight fists.

2. Open your hands and extend the
fingers.

3. Spread the fingers as far apart as you can.

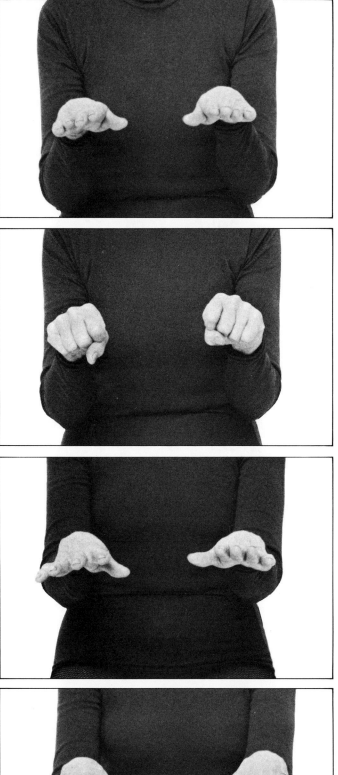

Do exercise 10 times.

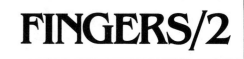

Starting Position: Turn the palm of your hand up, with fingers extended.

Movements:

1. Bring the little finger down to touch the palm, then lift it back up.

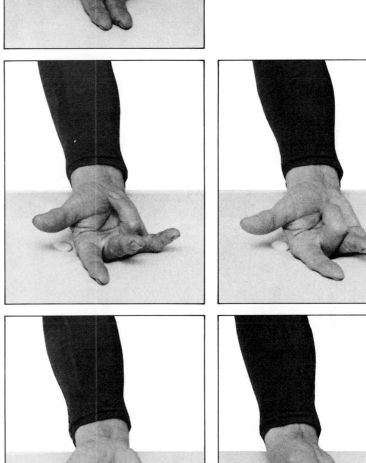

2. Repeat movements with ring finger.

3. Repeat movements with middle finger.

4. Repeat movements with index finger.

5. Now bring the thumb all the way across the palm to touch the pad of the little finger, then return it to its starting position.

Do exercise 2 times, then repeat exercise with the other hand, or do both hands at the same time.

FINGERS/3

Starting Position: Place your hands on a flat surface, palms down.

Movements:

Lift and lower one finger at a time. Do it 10 times before exercising the next finger.

Exercise all the fingers and then the thumbs in this manner.

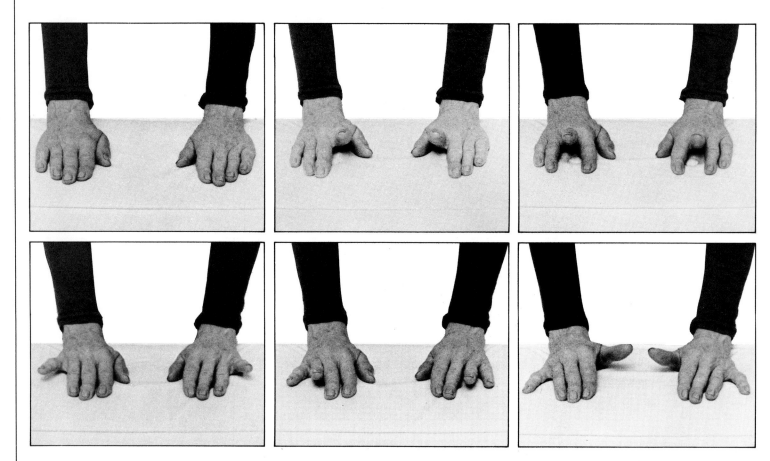

Do exercise once.

Starting Position: Place your hands on a flat surface, palms down. Bring fingers together to touch one another.

Movements:

1. Holding the other fingers steady, move the little fingers to the side.

2. Move the ring fingers toward the little fingers.

3. Bring the middle fingers toward the ring fingers.

4. Bring the index fingers toward the middle fingers.

5. Bring the thumbs toward the index fingers.

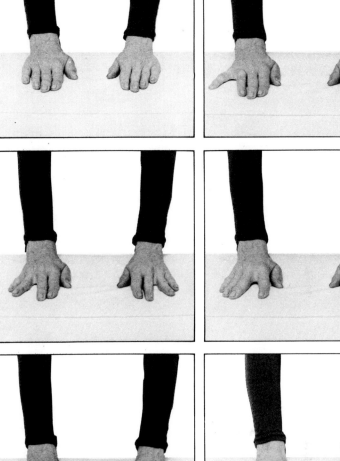

Do exercise 5 times.

FINGERS/5

Starting Position: Place your hands on a flat surface, palms down.

Movements:

1. Lift thumbs from the table and move them away from the index fingers.

2. Then move them back to touch the index fingers. Move the thumbs back and forth 5 times.

3. Spread the thumbs away from the fingers and place them back on the table.

Continue to move each of the other fingers out, and then back and forth, until you have exercised all of them.

Do exercise 2 times.

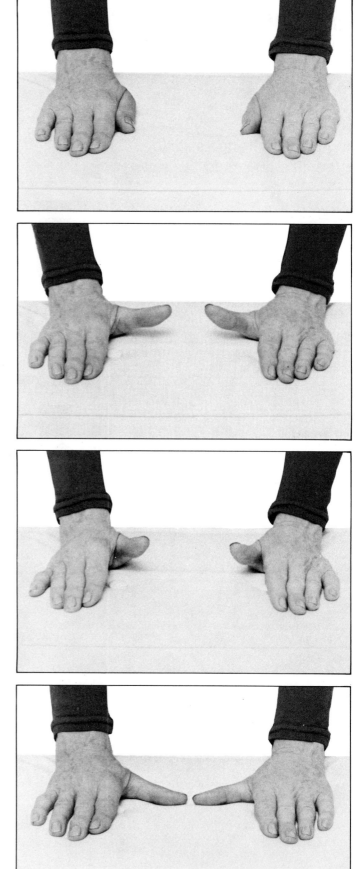

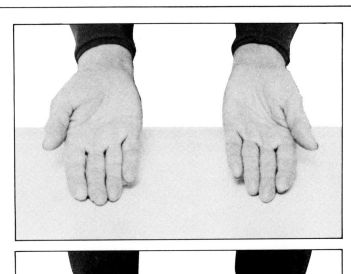

Starting Position: Put your hands out in front of you with the palms facing up.

Movements:

1. Bend the fingers down so that the tips touch the heels of your hands.

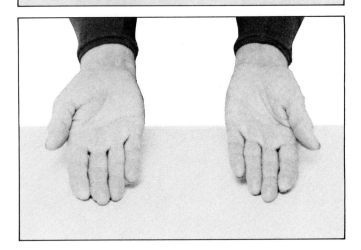

2. Extend your fingers.

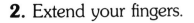

Bend and extend the fingers 20 times.

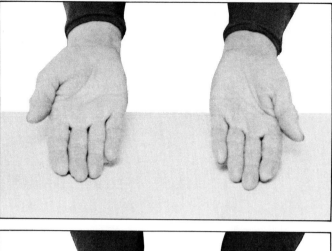

Starting Position: Turn your hands so the palms face up.

Movements:

1. Keep the palms of the hands extended and bend the fingers so that the tips just touch the pads at the base of the fingers.

2. Extend the fingers to their starting position.

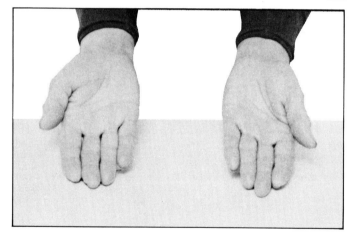

Close and extend the fingers 20 times.

Starting Position: Hold hands together, fingertips touching, in "tentlike" position.

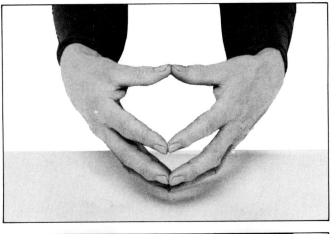

Movements:

1. Separate thumbs and circle them around each other; first circle 5 times toward the fingers, then reverse and circle 5 times in the other direction.

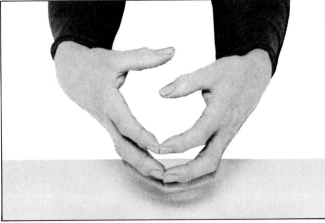

2. Touch thumbs to each other again.

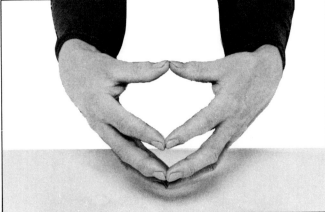

3. Now separate only the index fingers, and circle them around each other, first in one direction and then in the other.

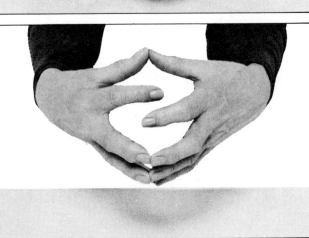

Circle the other three fingers in the same manner.

Do exercise once.

KNEES

The muscles that bend and straighten the knee are located in the front and back of the thigh. They work together with muscles of the hip and lower leg, thus permitting the knee to be bent and straightened in many different positions. Curiously, when walking, one uses the hip muscles more than those that bend the knee. In running, one bends the knee to a greater extent, but still not to its muscles' fullest capability.

Lack of use causes the knee-bending and -straightening muscles to become weakened, resulting in stiffened knee joints.

The following exercises have been designed to take the knee muscles through all their natural movements and tone the areas around the kneecap where fat gathers when muscles are not fully used.

KNEES/1

Starting Position: Sit in a straight-backed chair with your knees bent over the edge of the seat.

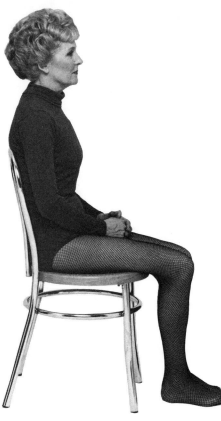

Movements:

Raise both legs, straightening the knees, and bring your feet parallel to the chair's edge.

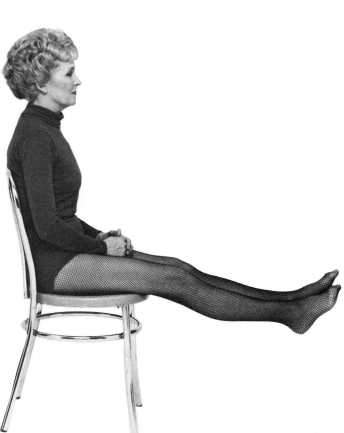

Straighten and bend your knees 20 times.

Starting Position: Stand with your side to the back of a chair, with your hands resting on it.

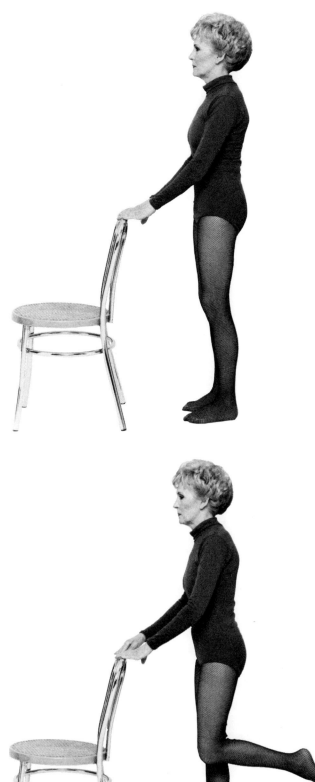

Movements:

Raise the left foot toward your buttock. Keep your back straight so that all the movement comes from the knee joint, not the hip joint.

Reverse sides and do the same exercise with the other leg, i.e., move the foot toward the buttock without bending your back.

Raise and lower each leg 20 times.

KNEES/3

Starting Position: Stand with your
right hand resting on the back of a
chair. Lift your left leg in front of you
by bending the knee.

Movements:

1. Point your toes toward the ceiling. Keep them in this pointed position and
bend and straighten your knee 10 times.

98

2. Now point your toes toward the floor. Keep them in this pointed position and again bend and straighten your knee 10 times.

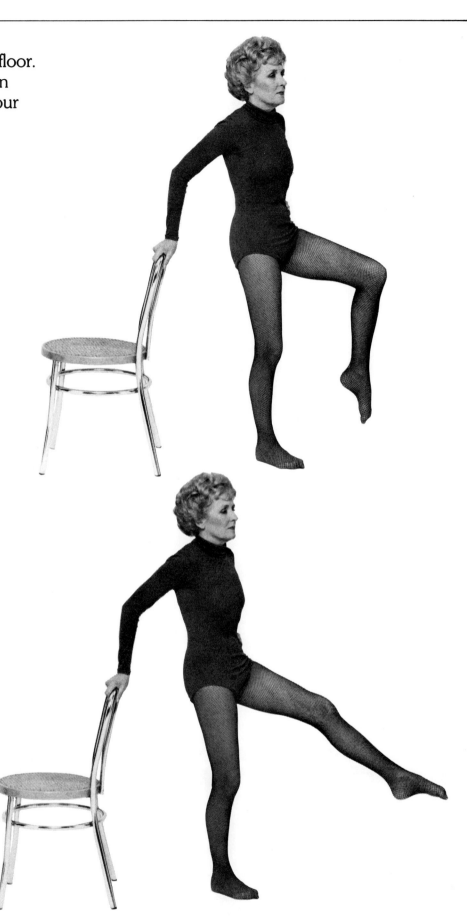

Do exercise 20 times. Then change legs and repeat with right leg.

Starting Position: Stand with both
hands resting on the back of a chair.

Movements:

1. Rise up on toes and bend your knees to bring the body to a squat
position. Hold for the count of 10.

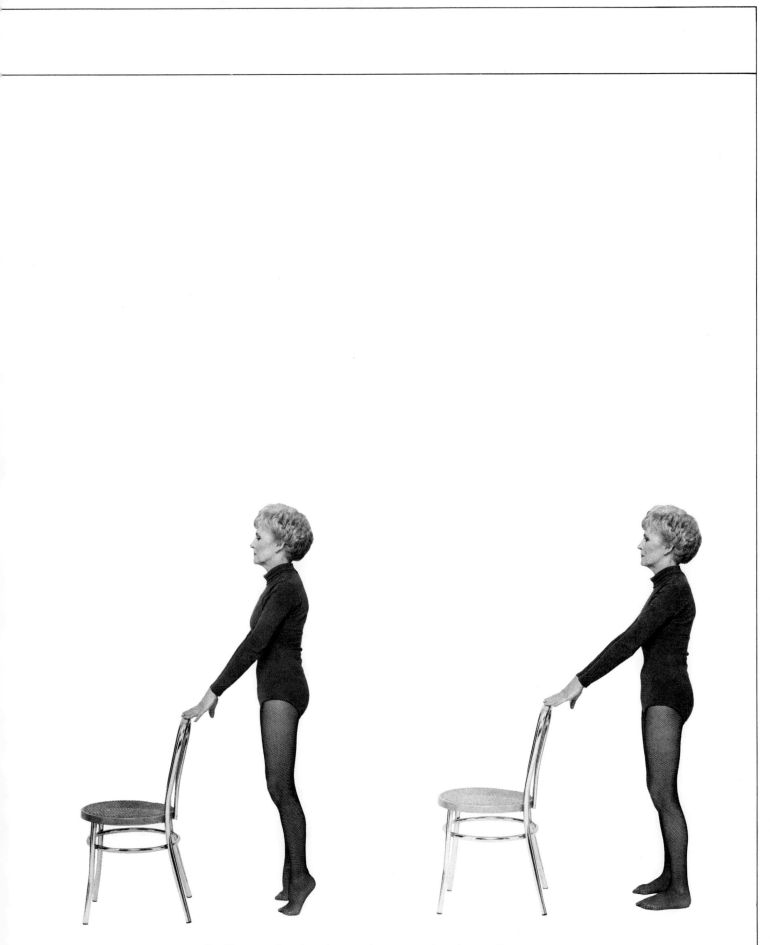

2. Raise the body and return heels to floor.

Do exercise 5 times.

KNEES/5

Starting Position: Hold on to a chair back with both hands. Bend the knees and bring your body to a kneeling position.

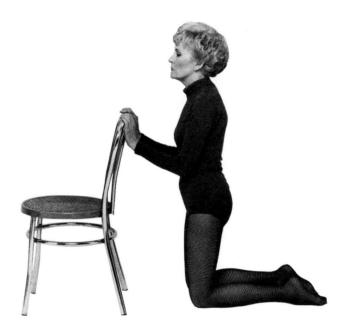

Movements:

1. Sit back on your heels.

2. Raise back up to your knees.

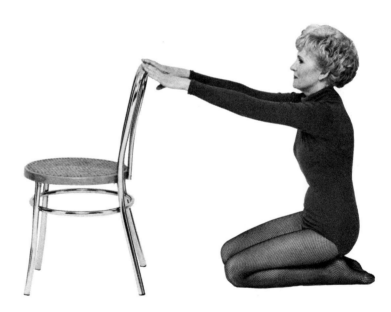

Sit and kneel 10 times.

Starting Position: Stand with your right hand resting on the back of a chair. Bend the left knee and place your foot on the side of your right knee.

Movements:

1. With the knee turned outward, straighten your leg.

2. Bend and straighten the knee without touching the foot to the floor.

Do exercise 20 times. Turn and do the same exercise with the right leg.

Starting Position: Stand with your
right hand on the back of a chair.
Turn the left foot outward. Place the
toes of your right foot directly behind
your left heel.

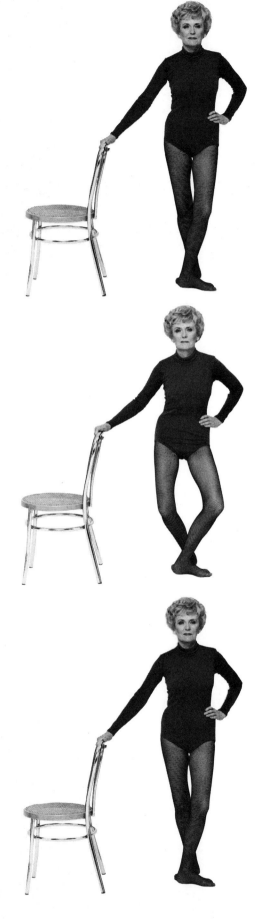

Movements:

1. Keeping the feet in the starting
position, bend your knees.

2. Straighten the knees.

Do exercise 10 times. Then change
position of right and left
feet and do 10 more times.

Starting Position: Stand with your right hand on the back of a chair. Bend the knee of your left leg and raise it in front of you.

Movements:

1. Keep the left foot totally relaxed, and make circles with the leg from the knee joint.

2. Circle leg 10 times to the right, then 10 times to the left.

Turn and repeat circling with the other leg.

LOWER BACK

Backache is often centered in the lower back. Weak muscles of the abdomen, the hips, the pelvic girdle, the ankles and arches and the spine are often the culprits that bring on lower-back pain. Excessive body weight can also cause back pain. Strengthening the muscles is your best insurance against suffering from a lower-back "condition."

These exercises for the lower back concentrate on using the back's "helping" muscles. If you want to do more, turn to the "Abdomen" and "Posture" sections.

When lifting heavy items, always bend the knees. Bended knees automatically force the thigh muscles to share the back's load.

LOWER BACK/1

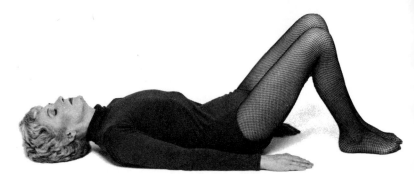

Starting Position: Lie flat on your back with knees bent and feet on the floor close to your buttocks.

Movements:

1. Slowly bring the right knee up, using your hands to pull it as close as possible to your chest.

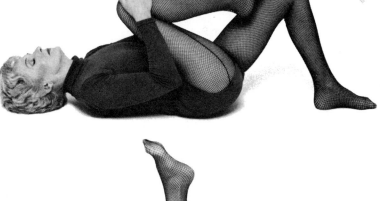

2. Straighten the leg and slowly lower it to the floor.

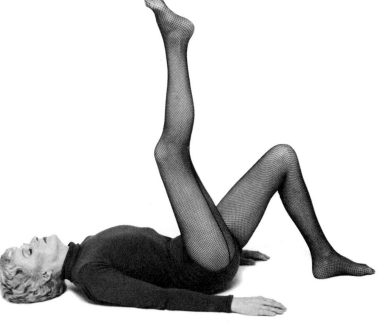

3. Bend the knee and bring the leg back to its starting position.

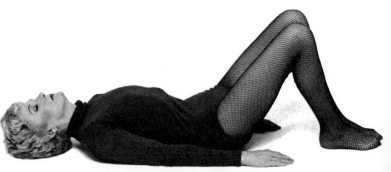

Do exercise 10 times.
Then repeat same movements with left leg.

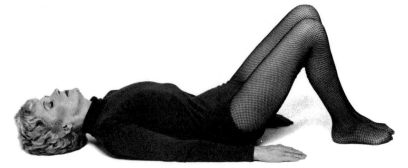

Starting Position: Lie flat on your back with knees bent and feet on the floor close to your buttocks.

Movements:

1. Bring your knees up toward your chest.

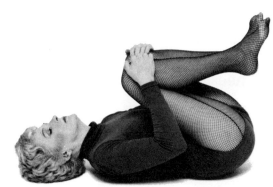

2. With both hands, pull the knees as close as possible to your chest.

3. Lift your head up as if to kiss your knees.

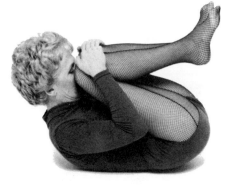

Do exercise 10 times.

(At first you may not be able to bring your knees to your head, but in time you will.)

LOWER BACK/3

Starting Position: Get down on your knees and rest the top of your head on your forearms.

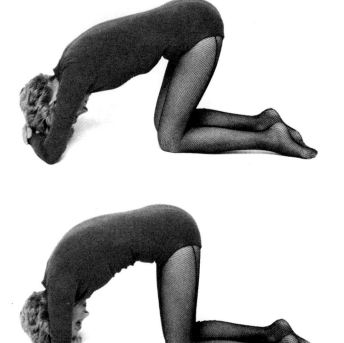

Movements:

1. Pull your stomach in.

2. Curve your back.

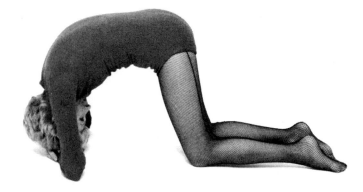

3. Keeping the back curved and stomach pulled in, roll your body forward on your knees.

4. Hold the body in this stretched position for a second.

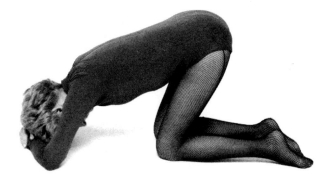

5. Roll back and relax the stomach muscles.

Do exercise 10 times.

Starting Position: Squat on your
toes, holding on to the seat of a chair
for support.

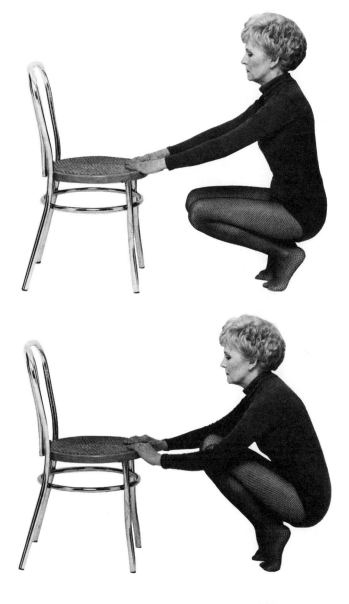

Movements:

1. Bring the knees up to the chest.

2. Return knees to starting position.

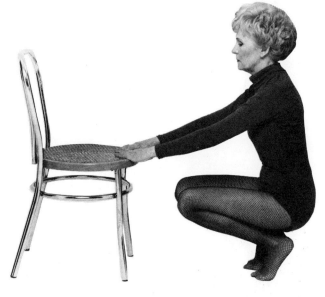

Do exercise 10 times.

LOWER BACK/5

Starting Position: Sit on the floor with your back flat against the wall—knees bent and heels touching, feet splayed outward.

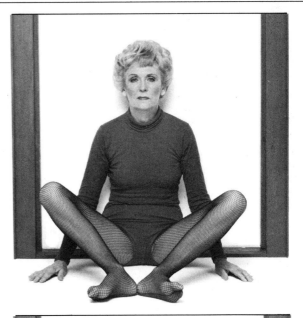

Movements:

1. Pull stomach in, and at the same time arch your feet by pointing the toes and bringing the soles of your feet toward each other.

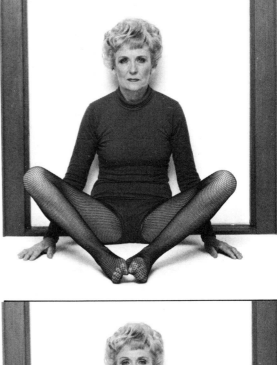

2. Relax stomach and return feet to the starting position.

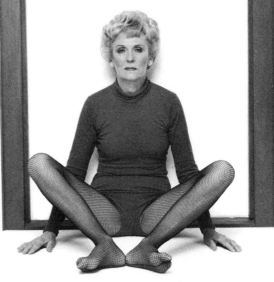

Do exercise 10 times.

Starting Position: Sit on the edge of a straight-backed chair with feet resting flat on the floor and hands on your knees.

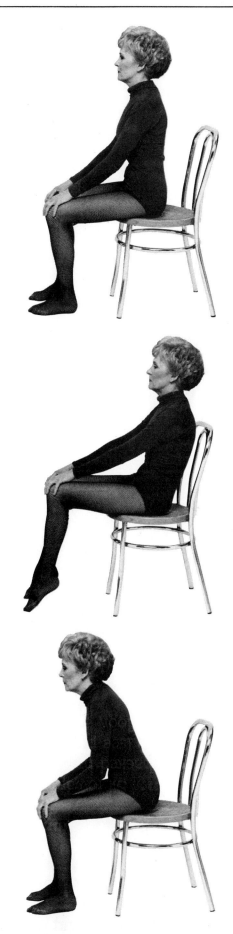

Movements:

1. Come up on your toes and roll backward on your buttocks, pulling stomach in as you do so.

2. Bring heels down to the floor. Relax stomach muscles. Roll forward on your buttocks and bring the torso back up to a straight position.

Using abdomen and back muscles, keep rolling back and forth, creating almost a "rocking-chair" motion.

Do exercise 20 times.

LOWER BACK/7

Starting Position: Stand with feet in a "lunge" position, putting the left leg well in front of the right. Raise right arm above your head.

Movements:

1. Shift your weight to the right leg so that your arm and head automatically go back.

2. Shift your weight forward to bring your head and arm forward.

3. Shift your weight back and forward 10 times.

Now put the left foot forward and repeat exercise 10 times.

Starting Position: Stand with your back to a doorjamb, with feet about 16 inches from it and slightly separated.

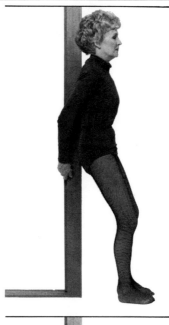

Movements:

1. Bend the knees and slide down the wall so that you are almost in a sitting position. Press the small of the back against the wall.

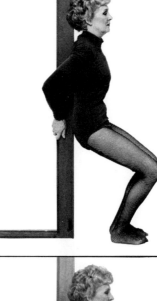

2. Slowly slide up, pushing the small of the back against the wall and straightening your knees as you do so.

Hold the upright position for a few seconds, then slide down the wall again.

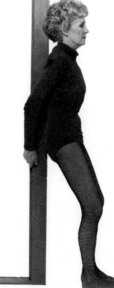

Do exercise 10 times

NECK

The muscles at the back of the neck restore the head to its erect position, after it has been drawn backward. They also serve to flex, rotate and turn the face from side to side. When these muscles weaken because of lack of use, gravity tends to bring the head forward and down toward the chest. Tension seems to concentrate at the back of the neck because rarely does one move the head as much as should be done. Probably one of the greatest signs of aging is the condition of the neck. The exercises in this section have been designed to help lengthen the neck by strengthening the muscles that hold it in an erect position (which means it will also look less thick); they also will foster greater mobility of the neck and improve the area where the neck joins with the chin and causes it to appear "double."

NECK/1

Starting Position: Stand with your chin resting on your chest.

Movements:

1. Keeping chin pressed to your chest, turn your face toward the right shoulder.

2. Still keeping chin pressed to the chest, roll your head toward the left shoulder.

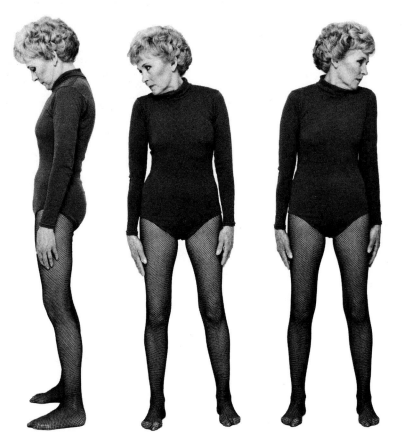

Repeat the exercise, bringing your head to the right shoulder and then to the left—like the movement of a windshield wiper. Do exercise 20 times.

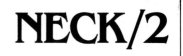

Starting Position: Stand and let your head fall back as far as it will go.

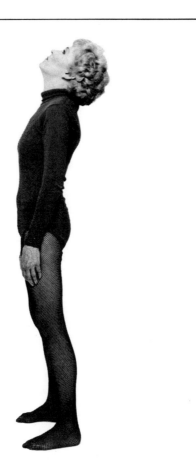

Movements:

1. From this position, without moving the shoulders, turn your head and look over your right shoulder.

2. Turn head back to starting position.

3. Without moving the shoulders, turn your head to look over your left shoulder.

4. Bring your head back to its normal position and relax.

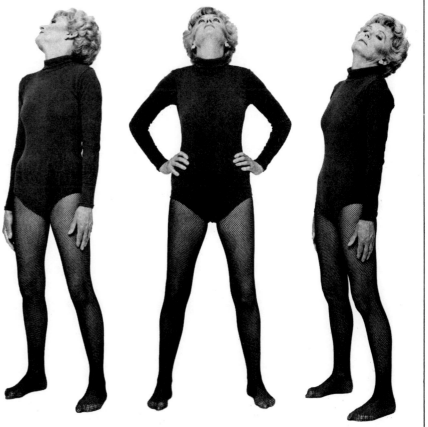

Do exercise 10 times.

Starting Position: Let your head fall over to the right shoulder as though you were slowly falling asleep.

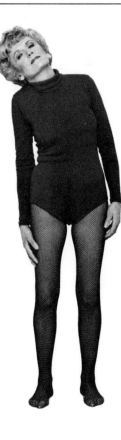

Movements:

1. Bring head back to an erect position.

2. Now let your head nod off to the left shoulder. Let it fall in little bounces—as slowly as possible.

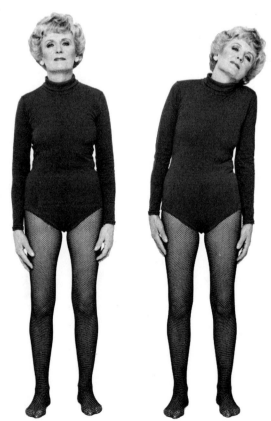

Do exercise 5 times on each side.

Starting Position: Rest your ear on the right shoulder.

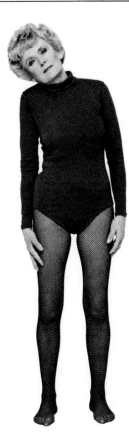

Movements:

1. Keeping your head in this position, bring chin toward chest.

2. Raise chin away from chest.

3. Drop the left ear to your shoulder and repeat the action.

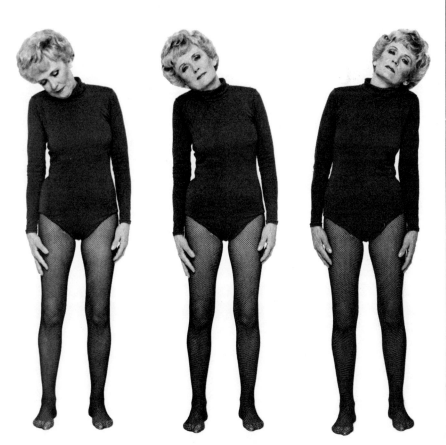

Do exercise 8 times on each side.

NECK/5

Starting Position: Stand with your head held erect.

Movements:

1. Move your head down and rest your ear on the right shoulder.

2. Keeping your head as close to the shoulder as you can, roll your head backward toward your center back so that you are looking at the ceiling directly overhead.

3. Now rest your head on the left shoulder and repeat movements.

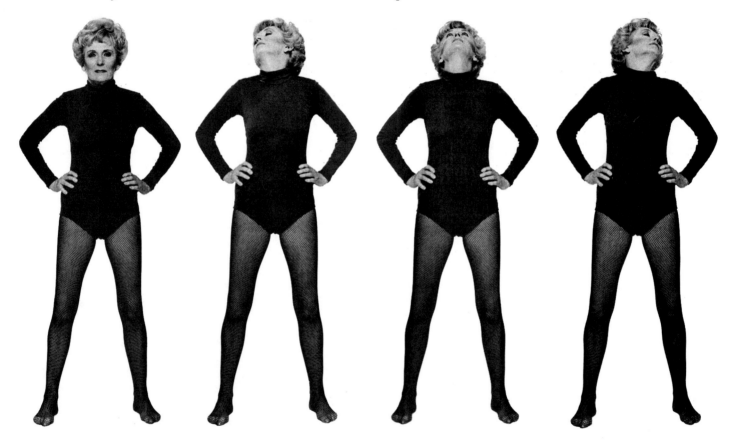

Do exercise 8 times.

Starting Position: Stand with head and shoulders erect.

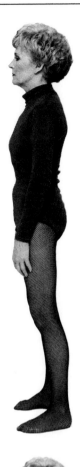

Movements:

1. Keeping the head's "fixed" position, move chin forward as far as you can.

2. Return it to starting position.

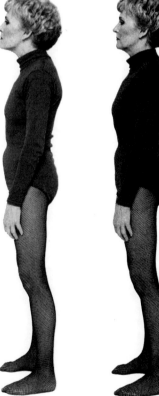

Do exercise 10 times.

NECK/7

Starting Position: Hold head and shoulders erect.

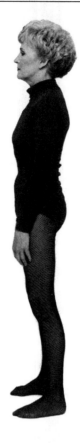

Movements:

1. Keeping the head's "fixed" position, move chin backward as far as you can.

2. Return it to starting position.

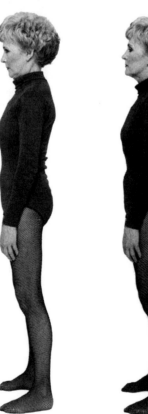

Do exercise 10 times.

Starting Position: Hold head and
shoulders erect.

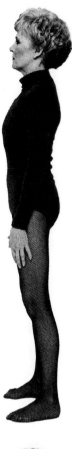

Movements:

1. Hold the head in a rigid position and
move the neck and head column slightly
backward.

2. Return it to starting position.

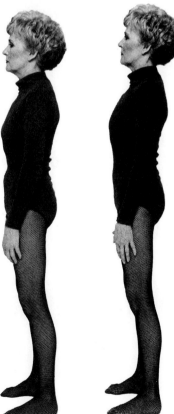

Do exercise 10 times.

POSTURE

The positions which you assume as you sit or stand can account for the body's being "in" or "out" of shape, since they affect the muscles that contour the body. For example, incorrect posture often results in protruding abdomens (polite words for potbelly), rounded shoulders, sagging bosoms and chests, a lump at the back of the neck euphemistically known as the "dowager's hump"—though many men, as well as women, have this disfigurement, which is caused by weakened neck and shoulder muscles that cause the head to be thrust forward in a dropped position. It is important to do exercises that specifically help strengthen these weakened muscles, but since everyone sits and stands for much longer periods than they exercise, it is equally important, as a preventive measure, to learn how to sit and stand correctly.

The following group of exercises is designed, therefore, to help you not only to get but to keep all the muscles of the body in tone while sitting and standing. Once you've learned them, bring them into play whenever you have to sit or stand for any long period of time.

To sit correctly, the trunk should rest on what is called the ischium, known familiarly as the "sit bones."

TO LOCATE SIT BONES

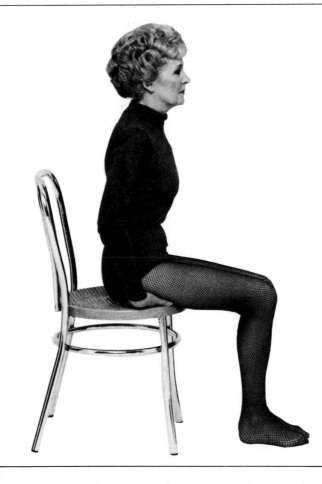

To locate the "sit bones," *sit toward the edge of a straight-backed hard chair. Put both hands beneath your buttocks, then rock your body from side to side until you feel a bone; that is the ischium. Every time you sit in balance on the ischium (as you will learn to do in the following simple exercises), you will be bringing tone to the abdominal muscles.*

POSTURE/1

To Help Reduce Midriff Section

Starting Position: Sit toward the edge of a straight-backed hard chair on your "sit bones" (see page 127), with feet flat on the floor, and arms at sides.

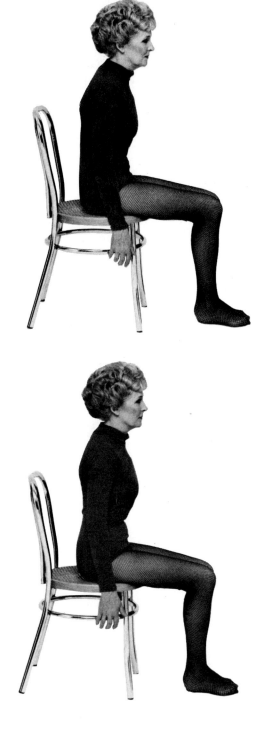

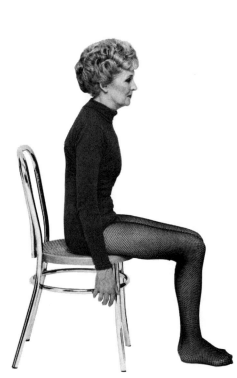

Movements:

1. Press your weight down.

2. Pull stomach muscles in and lift your chest up to straighten the spine.

Do exercise 10 times. But more important—remember to sit in the erect position every opportunity you get.

To Help Reduce the Buttocks

Starting Position: Sit on your "sit bones" (see page 127), with feet flat on the floor, arms at sides.

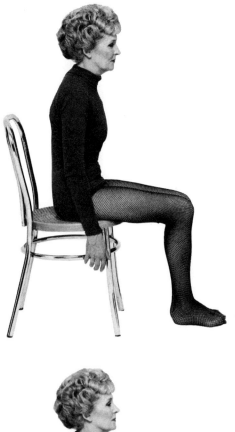

Movements:

1. Raise your chest to straighten the spine, press your weight down and press your thighs together as tightly as you can.

2. Relax thighs and buttocks.

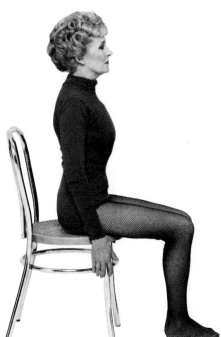

Do 20 times, or as often as you like.

POSTURE/3

To Help Reduce the Upper Back

Starting Position: Sit toward the edge of a chair, balancing on your "sit bones" (see page 127), with feet flat on the floor, arms at sides.

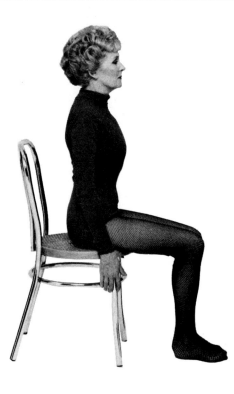

Movements:

1. Press your weight down and bring your chest up to straighten the spine. Hold that position.

2. Squeeze your shoulder blades together.

3. Relax.

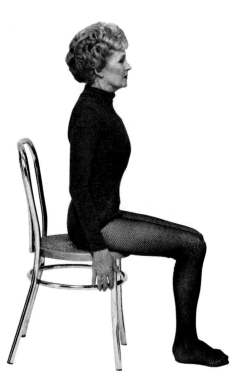

Do at least 10 times for every hour you sit.

To Help Prevent or Alleviate "Dowager's Hump"

Starting Position: Sit toward the edge of a chair on your "sit bones" (see page 127), with feet flat on the floor, arms at sides.

Movements:

1. Bring your chest up to straighten the spine. Hold your spine erect. Lift your chin and hold your neck erect.

2. Holding this position, push your neck backward to line up with the spine. (When done correctly, you will feel the movement in the "dowager hump" area.)

Do exercise 10 times.

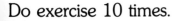

POSTURE/5

To Help Prevent and to Alleviate Lumps and Bumps on the Entire Body

Incorrect posture creates protruding abdomens, thick waistlines, rounded shoulders and double chins.

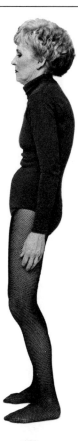

Starting Position: Stand with your feet together, arms at your sides.

Movements:

1. Lift your chest up to bring spine into an erect position.

2. Hold spine erect and lift stomach muscles upward as if tightening a belt.

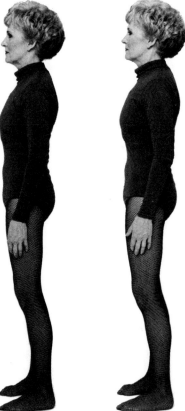

Do this exercise 10 times, and every time you find yourself just standing around. Always hold the muscles upward as long as you can.

To Help Firm the Buttocks

Starting Position: Stand with your feet about 6 inches apart and firmly planted on the floor. Place both hands on your buttocks to feel muscle movement.

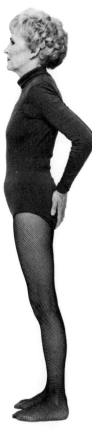

Movements:

1. Squeeze the buttocks together.

2. Bend knees slightly and pull stomach in, then squeeze the buttocks together even harder.

3. Relax the squeeze.

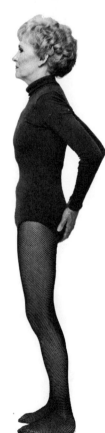

Do exercise 10 times, and every opportunity you have.

POSTURE/7

To Help Prevent and Alleviate "Dowager's Hump"

Starting Position: Stand with
knees bent so that the small of your
back is flat against the wall.

Movements:

1. Keeping this position, try to touch the
wall with the back of your head.

2. Still keeping back pressed to wall,
bring head forward.

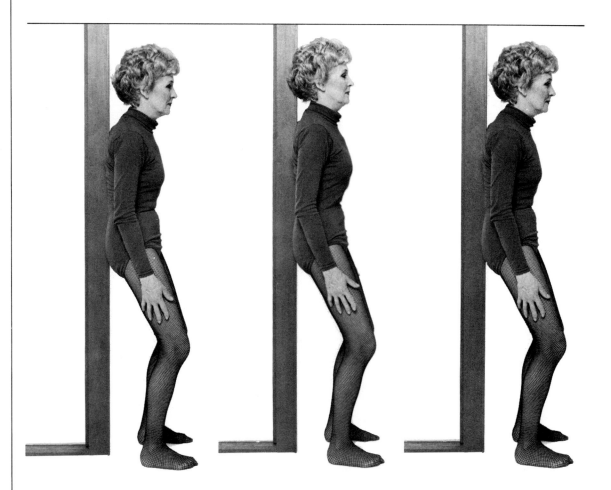

Do exercise 10 times.

Beneficial for Abdomen, Buttocks, "Dowager's Hump" and Upper Back

Starting Position: Stand with feet away from the wall, knees bent, and the small of the back and the base of the skull touching the wall. Keep torso and head pressed against the wall throughout exercise.

Movements:

1. Slide down the wall as far as you can.

2. Slide up the wall.

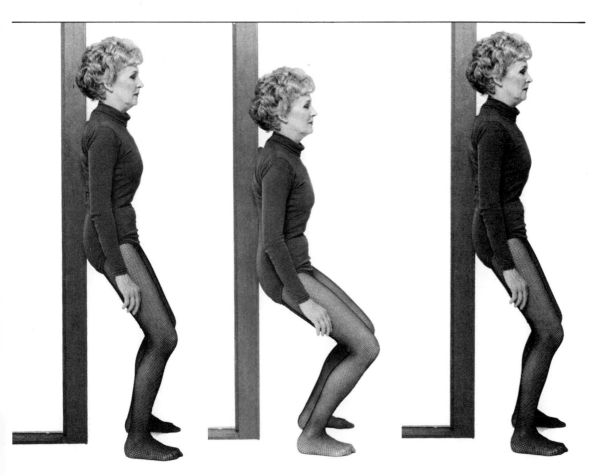

Do exercise 10 times.

SHOULDERS AND UPPER BACK

One of the dead giveaways of advancing age is a rounded upper back, which probably begins with a teen-age slump and increases with occupational postures, such as leaning over a desk or counter all day.

The muscles of the shoulders work together with those of the spine, neck, arms and chest. While lifting weights and doing other strenuous exercises can increase the size of the shoulders, the following exercises are intended only to tone the muscles of the shoulders and upper back, and thus to flatten the upper back. To maximize the benefits of these exercises, do the "Posture" exercises in conjunction with them.

SHOULDERS AND UPPER BACK/1

Starting Position: Stand with your hands on the back of a chair, head held naturally.

Movements:

1. Move your head directly backward so that it will rest on the upper back.

2. Fix the shoulders so they will not move, and push your head back even farther. Hold this position a second or two.

3. Slowly return head to starting position.

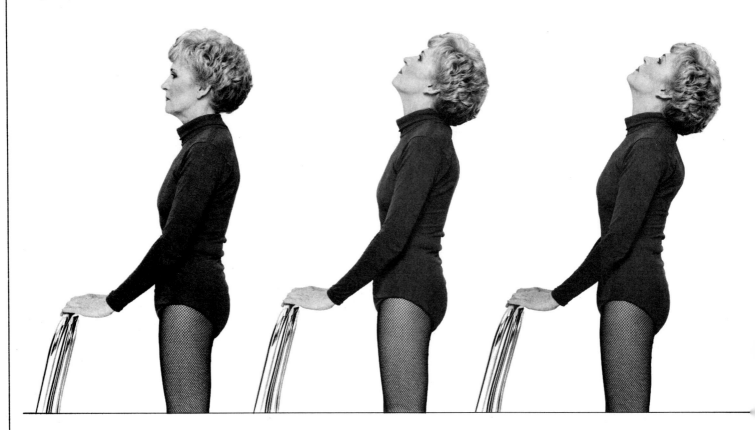

Do exercise 5 times.

Starting Position: Stand with hands on hips.

Movements:

1. Put your head back as far as you can and look up at the ceiling.

2. Keep that position, and turn your chin toward the right shoulder.

3. Continuing to look at the ceiling, bring your head back to center.

4. Still looking up, turn your chin toward the left shoulder.

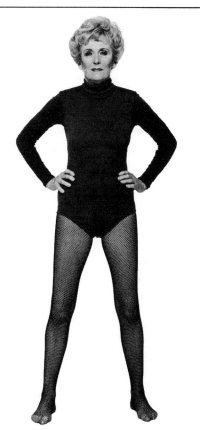

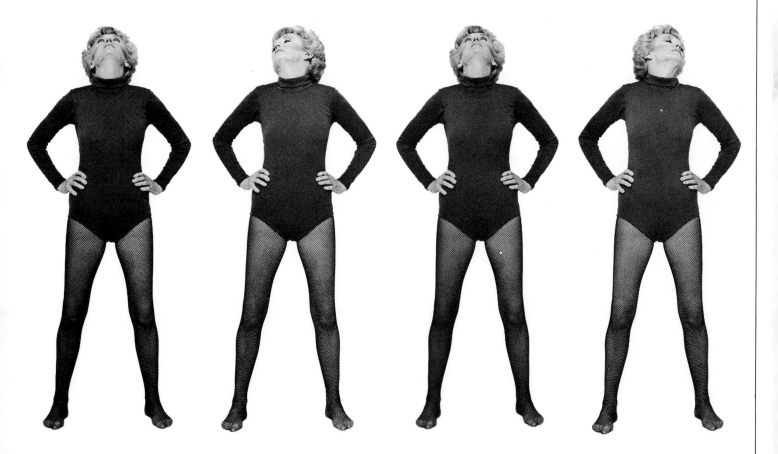

Do exercise 10 times.

Starting Position: Stand with the backs of your hands touching each other in front of your body.

Movements:

1. Swing your arms around and clap hands behind you.

2. Swing your arms to the front and bring the backs of your hands together.

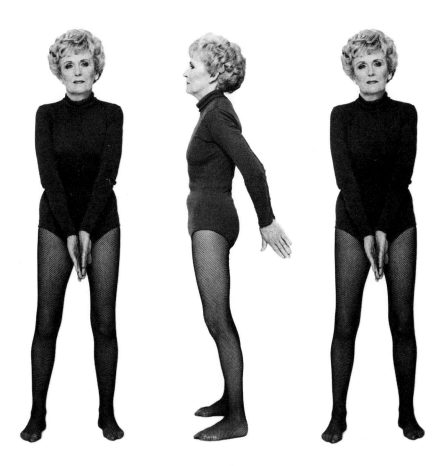

Do exercise 20 times.

Starting Position: Stand with arms held loosely at your sides.

Movements:

1. Move your shoulders up toward your ears.

2. Return them to their natural position.

3. Move your shoulders backward and squeeze blades together.

4. Return them to their natural position.

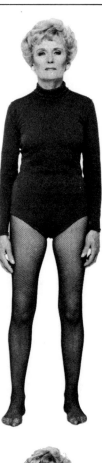

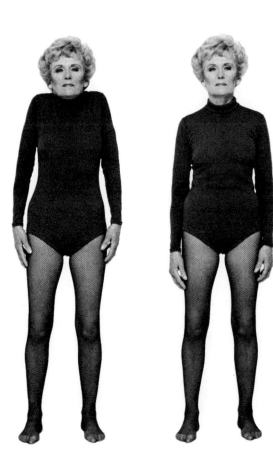

Do exercise 20 times.

Starting Position: Stand with feet firmly planted on the floor. Raise arms out to the side at shoulder level. Turn arms so that the backs of the hands face forward. Hold your hands in this position throughout the exercise.

Movements:

1. Bring arms forward to cross in front of your chest.

2. Return arms to starting position.

Do exercise 20 times.

Starting Position: Stand with hands in front of your chest, fingertips just touching.

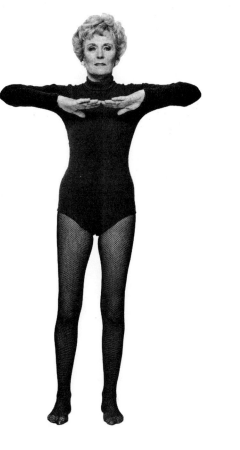

Movements:

1. Bring the elbows back to separate your hands and squeeze the shoulder blades together.

2. Return arms to starting position.

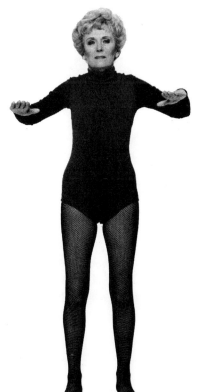

Do exercise 20 times.

SHOULDERS AND UPPER BACK/7

Starting Position: Stand with feet firmly planted on the floor, arms raised over your head, hands clasped.

Movements:

1. Keeping the hands clasped, move arms back behind your head.

2. Relax your shoulders, permitting the arms to return to starting position.

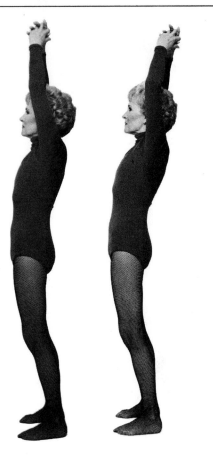

Do exercise 20 times.

Starting Position: Stand with arms raised over your head.

Movements:

1. Move arms backward and downward to start a circle.

2. Then, bring the arms forward and upward in front of the body to complete the circle.

Do exercise 20 times.

THIGHS

Thighs are thin, thighs are fat, the inner thigh sags, the outer thigh bulges, the back of the thigh becomes dimpled, the front of the thigh gets fat (it also sags). In other words, the thighs present a part of the body that non-exercisers like to keep covered.

The thigh muscles work jointly with those of the knee, calf, buttocks and hips. Often these latter muscles are used more than the thigh muscles themselves. Thigh muscles are intended to extend and bend the lower leg, to bring it outward and inward and to rotate the thigh inward and outward— movements rarely done in daily activities.

THIGHS/1

Starting Position: Lie face down on the floor with a pillow beneath the abdomen. Place your legs close to each other and bend the knees.

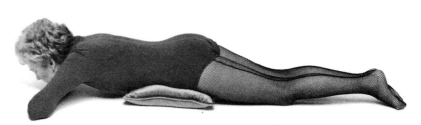

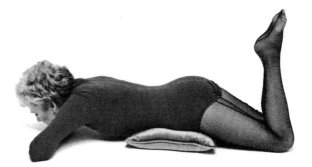

Movements:

1. Straighten and then bend the right leg.

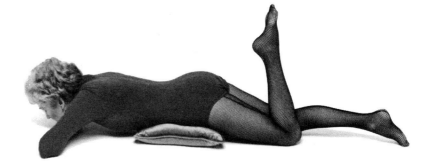

2. Straighten and then bend the left leg.

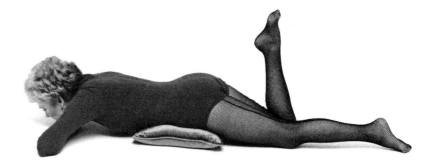

Alternate straightening and bending each leg. Do this as rapidly as you can 20 times.

Starting Position: Lie on the floor on your back, with knees bent over your torso and the soles of the feet touching.

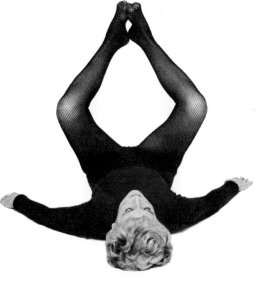

Movements:

1. Keeping this position, bring your knees together so that they touch.

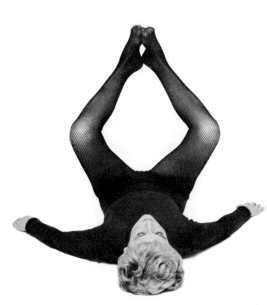

2. Still keeping the feet together, separate the knees as far apart as possible.

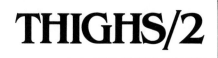

Do exercise 20 times.

THIGHS/3

Starting Position: Lie on the floor on your back, with legs extended over torso. Turn your feet inward until the tips of the toes touch.

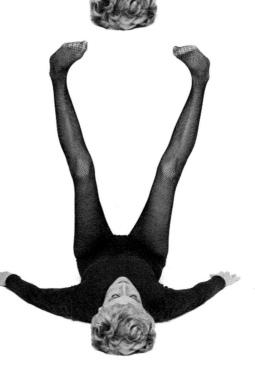

Movements:
Keep feet turned in this position and spread your legs apart as far as you can. Then bring them back to starting position.

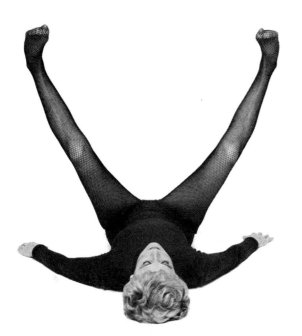

Do exercise 20 times.

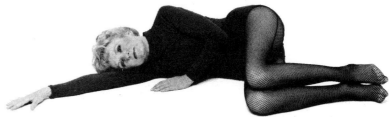

Starting Position: Lie on the floor on your right side, with knees pulled up high enough to make a lap, one leg lying on top of the other.

Movements:

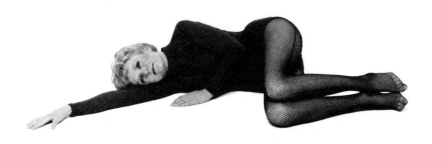

1. Bring the left knee as close to your chest as you can.

2. Return the knee to the starting position.

Bring left knee to chest 15 times. Then turn onto your left side and repeat exercise with right knee.

THIGHS/5

Starting Position: Lie on the floor with the left foot close to the buttocks. Extend the right leg and turn its foot outward. Keep the leg straight and the foot turned in this outward position throughout the exercise.

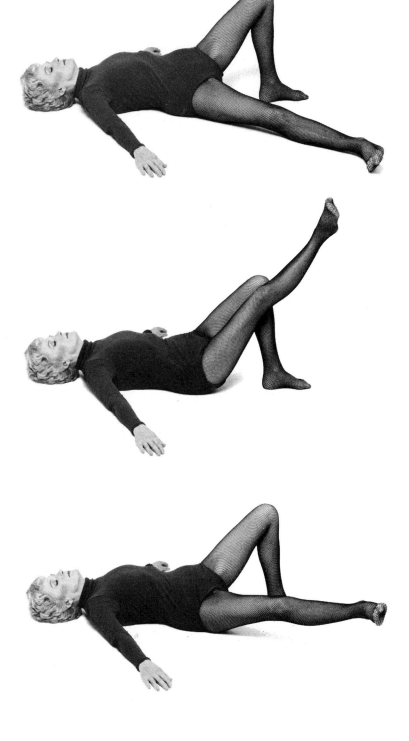

Movements:

1. Lift the right leg and touch its knee to the left knee.

2. Now move the leg as far away from the knee as you can without touching it to the floor.

Move leg toward and away from knee 15 times. Then do exercise 15 times with right knee bent and left leg straight.

Starting Position: Lie on your right side, with head resting on outstretched right arm. Keep the right leg straight and bend the left knee.

Movements:

1. Bring the bent knee across the straight leg and touch it to the floor.

2. Bring knee back to starting position.

Do exercise 20 times with left leg, then turn over and repeat exercise with right leg.

THIGHS/7

Starting Position: Stand with feet firmly on floor, knees slightly bent, legs about 16 inches apart, hands on hips.

Movements:

1. Move your knees toward each other. (Don't move your feet.) Bring them as close together as you can.

2. Return to starting position.

3. Move knees as far away from each other as you can.

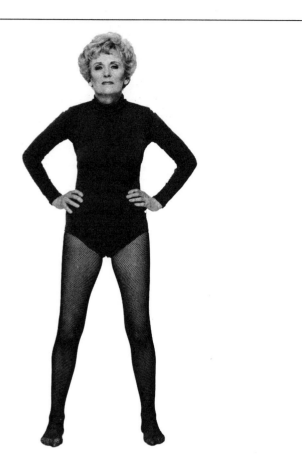

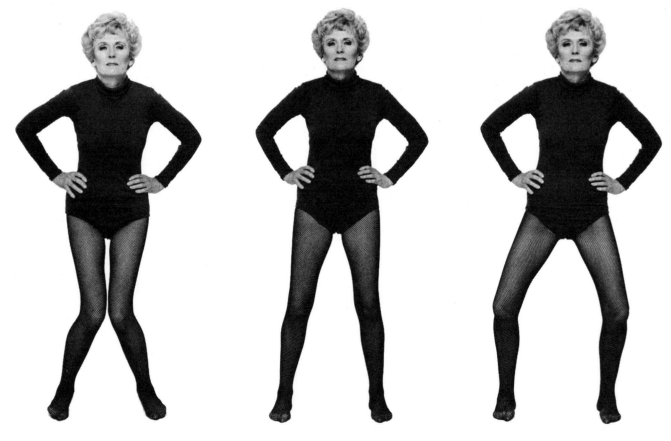

Do exercise 15 times. Do slowly for best results.

Starting Position: Stand with your back to a sturdy chair (far enough away from the chair to enable the top of the foot to rest on it when the knee is bent).

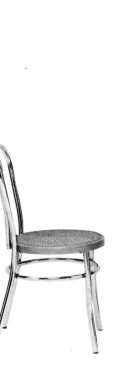

Movements:

1. Bend the right knee and rest your foot on the seat of the chair.

2. Return foot to floor.

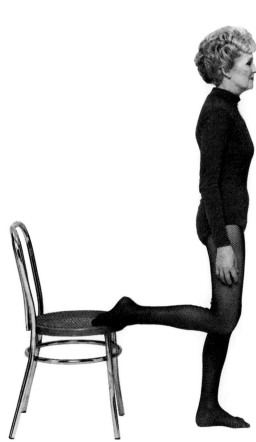

Do exercise 15 times with each leg.

WAISTLINE

The waistline separates the rib bones from the hip bones. If the ribs rest on the hips, bringing hips and ribs close together, it gives the figure the appearance of having a short, thick waistline. In olden days, a waistline was considered "whistle" material when it was ten inches less than the measurements of the bust and hips. Whatever size you seek for your waistline, the more distance you can put between the hip and rib bones will eventually be responsible for small, smaller, smallest measurement.

The waistline muscles are those that help to turn and twist the upper torso from side to side, bend it to the right and left sides and forward; they also work in conjunction with the diaphragm to aid in breathing. Toning these muscles helps to keep the waist wasplike, and also creates a "girdle" that smoothes away those ugly rolls and lumps that hang over belts.

(In preparing the manuscript of this section, I timed these exercises for one week—at the end of which I was staggered to discover that my waist measurement had decreased by more than an inch.)

WAISTLINE/1

Starting Position: Lie on your back on the floor, arms at your sides.

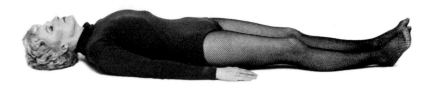

Movements:

1. Raise your head and shoulders from the floor. Hold that position and expel all the air from the lungs.

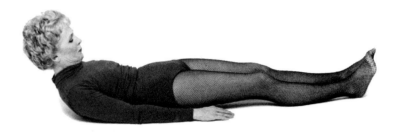

2. Breathe in, and return your head and shoulders to the floor.

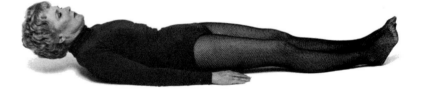

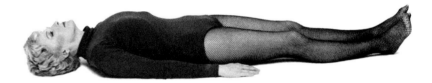

Do exercise 5 times.

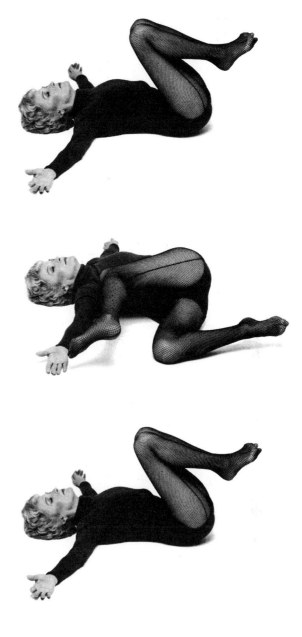

Starting Position: Lie on the floor on your back, arms extended out to the side at shoulder level. Bend knees toward the chest.

Movements:

1. Bring the left foot over your body and try to touch it to your right hand.

2. Roll back to the center position, and then touch the right foot to your left hand.

Do exercise 20 times.

WAISTLINE/3

Starting Position: Lie down on the floor on your right side, in a slightly crescent-shaped position, with your arms extended above your head.

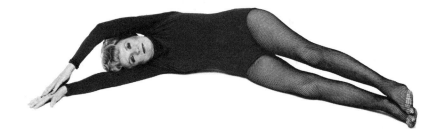

Movements:

1. Raise the torso and touch your thigh with your left hand.

2. Slowly lower body to starting position.

Do exercise 10 times on each side.

Starting Position: Stand with knees slightly bent, arms extended over your head.

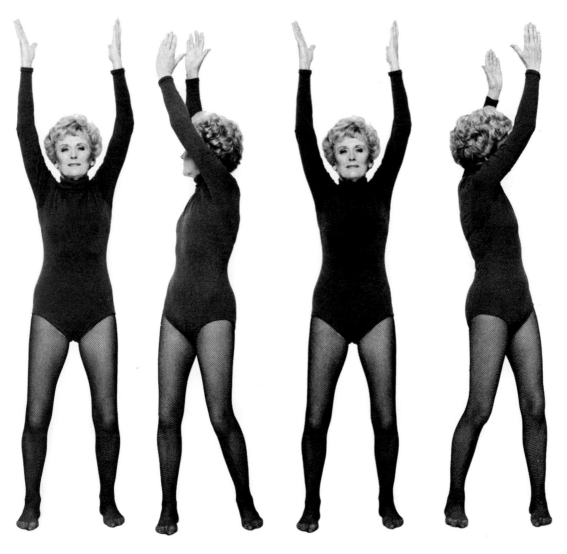

Movements:

1. As slowly as you can, twist the upper part of the body as far as possible to the right to look at the wall behind you.

2. Then twist, in the same manner, to the left.

Twist and turn to each side 20 times.

WAISTLINE/5

Starting Position: Stand with knees slightly bent, feet well separated and planted firmly on the floor. Clasp your hands behind your neck.

Movements:

1. Keeping this position, bend your body to the right side—as far as you can. Try to make your left elbow point directly up to the ceiling.

2. Bring body back to upright position.

3. Repeat the bending action to the left side of body.

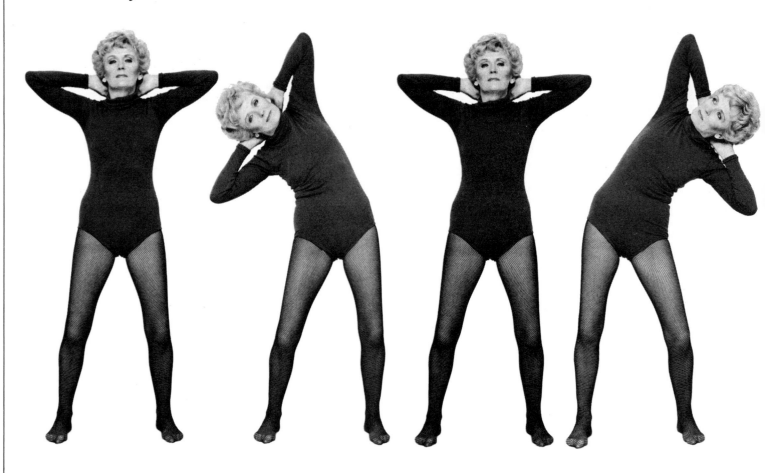

Do exercise 20 times.

Starting Position: Sit on a chair,
feet flat on the floor and well
separated. Put your hands together
and rest them on the right knee.

Movements:

1. Bending from the waist, slide your hands down to your toes.

2. Keeping the body bent and hands together, slide your hands along the floor to touch the toes of your left foot.

3. Slide your hands up to the left knee, straightening the body as you do so.

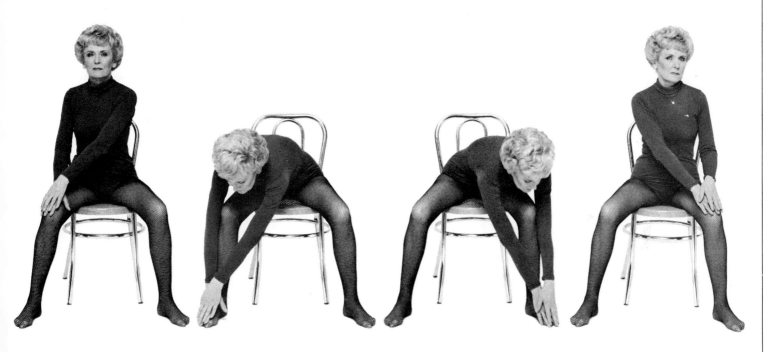

Do exercise 10 times. Then do 10 more times with hands starting on left knee.

WAISTLINE/7

Starting Position: Stand with right foot resting on the seat of a chair. Clasp your hands behind your neck.

Movements:

1. Bend at the waist and bring right elbow as close as you can to right knee.

2. Return to starting position.

3. Bend at the waist and bring left elbow as close as you can to right knee.

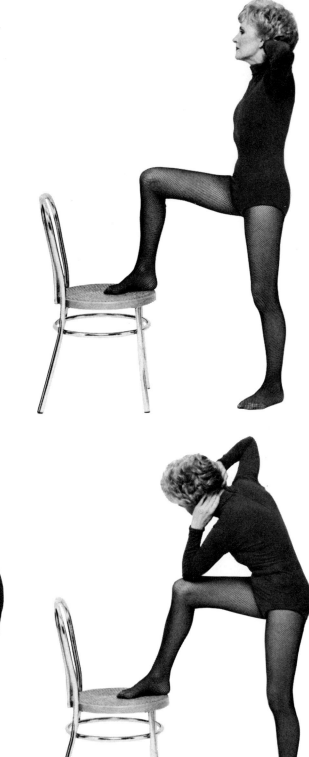

Do exercise 20 times. Rest left foot on chair and do 20 times more.

Starting Position: Bend your knees deeply and stand with the small of the back pressed against a wall, hands on thighs, feet firmly planted on the floor.

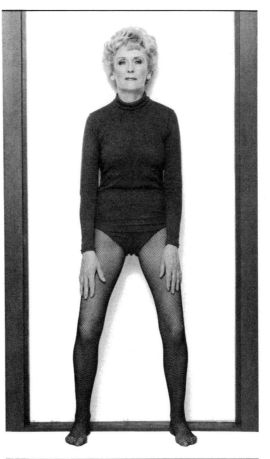

Movements:

1. Take a deep breath.

2. Bend at the waist and slide your hands down to touch the knees, keeping the small of your back pressed against the wall and expelling the air from your lungs as you bend.

3. Take a deep breath and bring body back up to starting position.

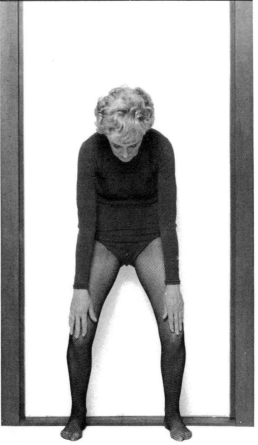

Do exercise 10 times.

WRISTS

The muscles of the wrist work in concert with those of the hands, fingers and forearms. Control of the wrist action quite often separates the good athletes from the bad. To control the action of the wrist and to strengthen and tone its muscles, its various capabilities must be brought into play. The wrist can be twisted, yes, but it also needs to be bent, turned and, certainly, straightened. The exercises in this section are almost guaranteed to allow you to deal with everything in sports with a flip of the wrist—provided, or course, you want to. But most assuredly they will strengthen the wrists, leaving up to you the skill with which you play.

WRISTS/1

Starting Position: Stand with arms alongside your body, wrists bent and fingers extended forward. Keeping the fingers in this position, move your arms out about 6 inches away from your body.

Movements:

1. Now turn the wrists so that the fingers point to the sides of your body.

2. Turn the wrists outward, and keep turning until your fingertips are pointing behind you.

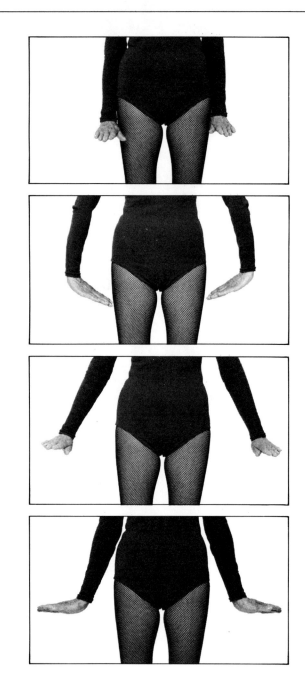

Do this circling motion 20 times.

Starting Position: With elbows bent and held close to the body, raise your forearms to waist level, hands turned down.

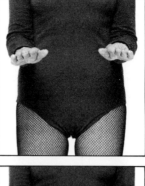

Movements:

1. Holding the elbows pressed to the body, bend your wrists and point your fingertips toward the floor.

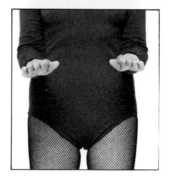

2. Slowly straighten the wrists and bring your hands to their starting position.

Do movements 20 times.

WRISTS/3

Starting Position: With elbows bent and held close to the body, raise your forearms to waist level, hands turned down.

Movements:
Holding the elbows pressed to your body, rotate your wrists to make your hands go around in circles.

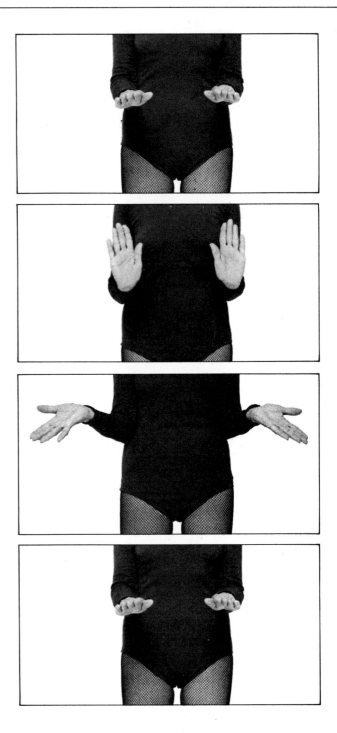

Circle in one direction 10 times. Then circle in opposite direction 10 times.

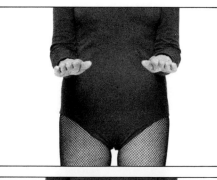

Starting Position: With elbows bent and held close to the body, raise your forearms to waist level, hands turned down.

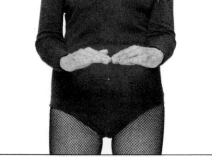

Movements:

1. Turn the wrists so that the fingertips point toward one another.

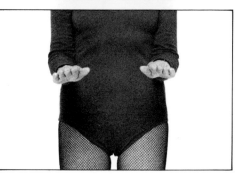

2. Slowly turn the wrists to bring the hands back to the starting position.

Do exercise 20 times.

WRISTS/5

Starting Position: With elbows
bent and held close to the body, raise
your forearms to waist level, hands
turned down.

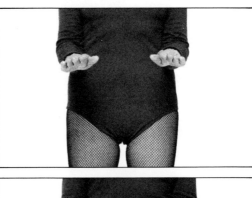

Movements:

1. Turn the wrists so that the fingers
point in an outward direction.

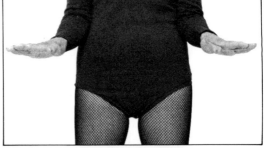

2. Slowly turn the wrists to bring the
hands back to the starting position.

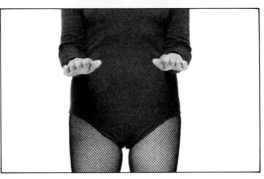

Do exercise 20 times.

Starting Position: Stand with the inner arms pressed to your body. Bend the elbows and bring the forearms to waist level, hands turned down. Now fold your fingertips so that they touch the heels of your hand.

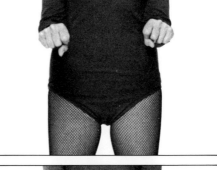

Movements:

1. Bend the wrists to move your folded hands in an outward direction.

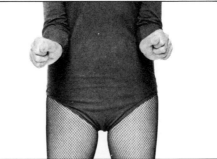

2. Bring wrists back to starting position.

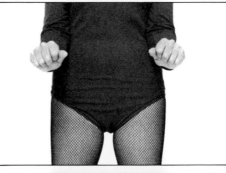

3. Move the wrists to bring the hands toward the body.

4. Bring wrists back to starting position.

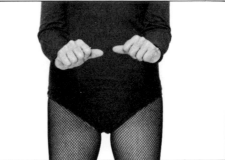

Do exercise 20 times.

WRISTS/7

Starting Position: With elbows bent and held close to the body, raise your forearms to waist level, hands turned down.

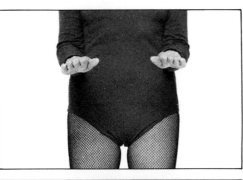

Movements:

1. Holding the elbows close to your body, bend your wrists so that your fingertips point toward the ceiling.

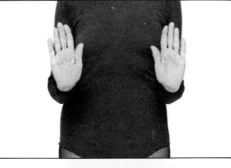

2. Slowly straighten the wrists and bring hands back to the starting position.

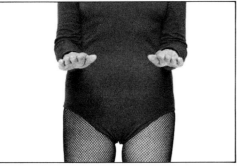

Do exercise 20 times.

Starting Position: With elbows bent, pressed to your sides, turn your palms up. Cup the palms, curving the fingers slightly upward. Hold the hands in this position throughout the exercise.

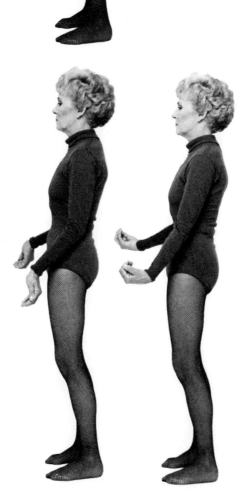

Movements:

1. Keeping the palms "cupped," slowly bend the wrists downward as far as they will go.

2. Slowly bend the wrists upward as far as they will go.

Do exercise 20 times.